# Transnational Social Support

# Routledge Studies in Health and Social Welfare

# Transnational Social Support

Edited by Adrienne Chambon, Wolfgang Schröer, and Cornelia Schweppe

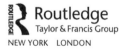
Routledge
Taylor & Francis Group

NEW YORK   LONDON

First published 2012
by Routledge
711 Third Avenue, New York, NY 10017

Simultaneously published in the UK
by Routledge
2 Park Square, Milton Park, Abingdon, Oxon OX14 4RN

*Routledge is an imprint of the Taylor & Francis Group,
an informa business*

Typeset in Sabon by IBT Global.

First issued in paperback 2013

*Library of Congress Cataloging-in-Publication Data*
   Transnational social support / edited by Adrienne Chambon, Wolfgang
Schröer, and Cornelia Schweppe.
      p. cm. — (Routledge studies in health and social welfare ; 7)
Includes bibliographical references and index.
   1. Social policy.   2. Social service.   I. Chambon, Adrienne S.,
1949–   II. Schröer, Wolfgang, 1967–   III. Schweppe, Cornelia, 1955–
   HN28.T698 2012
   361.2'6—dc23
   2011028076

ISBN13: 978-0-415-71972-8 (pbk)
ISBN13: 978-0-415-88876-9 (hbk)
ISBN13: 978-0-203-13941-7 (ebk)

# Contents

## PART III
## Transnational Family Care

## PART IV
## Transnational Social Support and Biography

## PART V
## Transnational Social Support: Unintended Consequences and
## Future Challenges

# Figures and Tables

## FIGURES

## TABLES

# 1 Introduction

*Adrienne Chambon, Wolfgang Schröer, and
Cornelia Schweppe*

Despite a wide range of theoretical and empirical analyses of the concept of transnationalism in the social sciences (sociology, political sciences, anthropology, economics, and geography), the notion has hardly been examined in a systematic fashion in social work with respect to the field's scholarly and professional developments (Homfeldt, Schröer, and Schweppe 2008; Negi and Furman 2010). Social work, as an applied professional field, can serve as a template for other professional disciplines such as education or nursing.

This volume focuses on social support from a transnational perspective and addresses a particular set of needs and the corresponding lack of appropriate responses. Social support indicates "the mechanisms through which a social environment protects its individual members from threatening and impairing events and experiences, and which can support them in their coping efforts" (Nestmann 2001: 1687). Social support encompasses measures, interventions, and social relationships that help ease burdensome and impairing life events, situations, or trajectories. Social support can further play a preventive role in promoting well-being and welfare.

In light of continually increasing mobility on a global scale, the challenges that social support will face in the future can no longer be addressed solely through the mechanisms, relationships, and structures of support shaped within national contexts. As a variety of studies *implicitly* show, transnationalism is associated with specific and manifold forms of social support. Yet, research that systematically locates transnational social support at the centre of analysis is just in its beginnings.

This publication addresses transnational social support from both a theoretical and an empirical research perspective. Its overall aim is to contribute to the introduction of a transnational perspective in the academic discipline and professional field of social work. Transnational approaches can extend and transform the conventional, nationally bounded approaches to both knowledge and practice. The aim is to incorporate a transnational dimension in the very knowledge structure of social work. The concept 'transnational social support' is a new entry point into social realities. It is located at the intersection between research on social support, social politics, and research on transnationality.

Different disciplines have adopted a wide range of meanings regarding the concept of transnationalism (Glick Schiller 1992; Faist 2000a, b; Levitt and Khagram 2007; Pries 2001, 2010; Vertovec 2009). New forms of compressed time and space have emerged against the background of growing globalisation, along with new developments in information technology and new modes of transportation. These changes include new forms of mobility and migration, and new forms of political, social, and economic cooperation in the context of social work. Recent research on transnational care already shows these new dimensions, but it has mainly concentrated on the transnational provision of care.

The term "global care chains" (Hochschild 2000) shows how the phenomenon is not a one-way process from poorer to richer countries. Thus, the Global Commission for Migration (2005) has pointed out that migration should be understood today as more of a circular process. Using this framework, it is possible not only to describe transnational processes of so-called 'brain circulation,' but also to observe processes of social support circulation. In the provision of care, the interconnection between the countries of origin and the destination countries has been analysed accordingly. Studies have traced forms of transnational motherhood and of family support structures in transnational sectors. And finally, attention has been paid to the working conditions of female transmigrants in different countries.

Transnationality[1] (or the conditions for transnationalism) is characterised by the circulation of people, goods, money, ideas, symbols, and cultural practices across traditional national reference points. In the process, new patterns emerge in terms of biography, space, and institutions. "A narrow understanding of the concept of *transnationalism* only refers to lasting, extensive, and institutionalised relationships that transcend national borders" (Pries 2002: 264, translation by the editors). Conceptualised more broadly, transnational patterns include feelings of belonging, common ideas and beliefs; the inextricability of economic, political, cultural, and social factors; connections in the labour force as well as relationships of dominance and their related organisational structures, which all transcend the borders of nation-states. Pries (2010) assumes a shared understanding about transnational processes: "In an expansive understanding of the concept, *transnationalism* refers to the sense of belonging, cultural commonalities, intertwined forms of communication, workplace contexts and everyday life practice, as well as to related social orders and regulations that transcend the borders of nation states" (3, translation by the editors). It is important to note that the concept of transnationalism does not deny the continued importance and relevance of nation-states (cf. Westwood and Phizacklea 2000). In contrast to the concept of globalisation, which focuses on the developments beyond nation-states, "research on transnational processes depicts transnational social relations as 'anchored in' while also transcending one or more nation-states" (Smith, quoted in Pries 2002: 7). Transnationality may be understood as a new context for social intertwining (Elias

1986) between the micro-level of social reality—the social dispositions and positioning of actors and their everyday life practice, their lifestyles, biographical projects, and identities—and the macro-level of social and political frameworks.

In taking a social actors approach, transnational social support can be understood as a social process of appropriating and designing social worlds across national borders, in which support activities are performed in either direct or indirect ways. *Based on our understanding of transnational social support as a social process, this publication will address it from individual, social, and political perspectives.*

The first section focuses on transnational social policy. The post–World War II welfare state (known as the Keynes-Beveridge model in the English-speaking world) was, at origin, a project of the nation-state. National boundaries were important because they identified eligibility for state benefits and offered an appropriate funding base. Recent years have called into question the relevance of a nation-state focus. The forces of globalisation foretold the decline of the nation-state. Governments within a traditional nation-state focus have been unwilling or incapable of providing this support within a transnational context.

Social policy, so far, has tended to emphasise links, activities, and processes occurring 'within' nation-states, to the neglect of those cutting across nation-states. This 'methodological nationalism' is increasingly being questioned as transnational processes have become more significant over the last half century. The spread of activities, links, and ties beyond national borders has become more extensive, and the interactions themselves have become more intensive.

The first section of the book will explore some of the ramifications for social policy, both conceptually and operationally, of a transnational world. It will re-examine mainstream social policy questions: Whose responsibility is it to deliver services in a transnational context? Who benefits? How and in what form? What is the role of the state and that of NGOs (including international NGOs)? Lightman, Böhnisch, and Schröer focus on these questions from two different perspectives.

Lightman analyses the challenges of transnational social policy from the perspective of migration. He embeds his analysis into an understanding of social policy, which refers to choices and options. Consequently, he understands transnational social policy as those choices that affect transnational migrants and the processes of transnational migration. Lightman contextualises his macro-level analysis within processes of globalisation and shows how these developments challenge the so-far nationally structured welfare state, and hence nationally bound social policy. He shows the close relationship between social policy and (trans)migration and analyses how (transnational) social policies have an important impact on the processes and outcomes of transmigration and vice versa. He also shows that transnational social policy is not just the inclusion of a new variable into social policy, but that it inevitably alters the calculus and the results. Lightman illustrates his chapter with examples mainly from Canada, but these are not less relevant to many other countries.

Böhnisch and Schröer approach transnational social policy from a different angle. They start from an analysis of the changing welfare state due to global developments. In the new governmental social order, previous state responsibility and its protective functions against social risks shift to conceptions that encourage self-responsibility of the individual and the activation of citizens. Asking about the future of the welfare state, the authors argue that going back to nationally bound states is no longer a viable perspective. The challenge is to look for a new balance instead, between the economic and the social, now against the background of transnationalised and globalised social structures. Within this context, Böhnisch and Schröer turn to the capability approach developed by Sen and Nussbaum and critically ask about its potential as a transnational platform of understanding. They reveal the capability approach as an unhistorical, decontextualised, and normative concept which is based on social anthropological assumptions of a 'good life.' They criticise the neglect of the analysis of the structural conditions of social needs and social risks which historically develop. Therefore, Böhnisch and Schröer plead for transnational social policy perspectives which are based on and rooted in the specific social historical development and structural conditions of the particular life conditions.

The second section of the book deals with transnational organisations and the question of how they shape transnational support processes. During the last twenty years there has been increasing attention devoted to transnational organisations that frame and provide social support and aid. Overall, transnational organisations increasingly produce knowledge and shape social and political developments that in turn have an impact upon the design of local and/or transnational support contexts. Within neo-institutional theories, these organisations are discussed primarily in terms of global governance (Kern 2004).

Transnational organisations seek to strengthen the agency of participating actors through expressed claims of self-legitimation. For instance, transnational organisations often explain their forms of social support and interventions as being informed by notions of empowerment or self-help. Additionally, they take up concepts of action from local grassroots movements (Sherraden and Ninacs 1998; McCall 2003) or foster the participation of actors in social and civil society development (Goetze 2002). Other authors, following Foucault's approach, argue that by focusing on agency, scholars tend to produce and reproduce precisely those norms—autonomy, self-determination, participation—through which the new governance has been structuring itself.

In this context, hopes are placed on a "global civil society" (Kaelble, Kirsch, and Schmidt-Gernig 2002) and on transnational non-governmental organisations (TNGO). TNGOs are still considered capable of providing considerable momentum to putting a human face on globalisation (Hofmann 2006: 179), but so far no common perspective regarding a global civil society is to be seen ('clash of definitions'). Furthermore, the growing linkage between TNGOs and other actors such as nation-states and confederations of nation-states (like the United Nations) is becoming subject to critical scrutiny (Frantz and Martens 2006: 86) with respect to the distribution of influence, power, resources, and staff in the TNGOs.

In their chapter, Ehlers and Wolff point out that a perspective of transnational organisational learning is necessary in the field of development cooperation. The debates about transnational organisations and development cooperation seem to be dominated by a normative and political attitude. Processes of organisational learning are not very often included in the view of a critical evaluation in this field. By analysing key situations and interactions, Ehlers and Wolff are able to show how organisations demonstrate their positions and simultaneously protect their own purpose. In the end it is obvious that people who organise transnational social support have to acquire a realistic view of the institutional and organisational arrangements.

The chapter by Smith also presents an inside view of transnational organisations. Based on ethnographic research in a transnational Japanese new religious movement, Sukyo Mahikari, Smith discusses these transnational organisations as providers of social support. In this perspective, Sukyo Mahikari is a professionally organised transnational stakeholder which offers social support through structures, rituals, and social activities for the members. Overall Smith argues that we have to analyse these organisations more deeply and critically because of their growing circulation and their importance for their members.

The third section of the book offers critical analyses of transnational family support, and each chapter brings a special focus on gender issues. Researchers in social support in the context of family relationships increasingly recognise the unique quantitative and qualitative dimensions of family and kin support, which stem from norms of mutual assistance and commitments to solidarity. In numerous studies, family and kin have turned out to be significant and reliable sources of support (Pierce, Sarason, and Sarason 1996). They effectively protect their members from harm to their well-being and contribute considerably to coping with crises. However, family social support can also result in considerable strain (Laireiter and Lettner 1993).

Good Gingrich raises very serious concerns about family support in the context of transnational migration. She examines the situation of the religious communities of Mennonite families migrating from Mexico to Canada, in light of the historical migration of these groups under the pressure of severe economic hardship and survival needs, and, in some cases, their pattern of return migration. The author's multiple studies show that the positioning of Mennonite family members and their mutual support system are imperilled in the context of the profound divergence of values between those they hold in their community of origin, and the labour, educational, and family priorities imposed upon them by the neo-liberal system that is dominant in Canada. The author characterises the existential situations of these families as an 'in-between' space faced with irreconcilable ways of being, in which the function and contribution of women is placed in severe jeopardy. This in-between-ness is the very nature of their difficulties. Institutional mechanisms of formal support, both professional and semi-professional, regrettably tend to reinforce these disjunctures and further contribute to the economic and symbolic violence exercised upon the women and their families as a result of migration.

Wang and Lin's chapter picks up the central practice of home care delivered by women migrants from more disadvantaged countries, and illustrates it with the case of Taiwan. Transnational family studies have important implications for understanding transnational forms of family social support. Since the end of the 1990s, research on systems of care has pointed to the growing transnationalisation of family assistance, nursing, and relationships of care as a global phenomenon. One example is the increasing transfer of assistance, nursing, and care services—performed mostly by women—from poor countries to the households of wealthier countries (Anderson 2000; Hondagneu-Sotelo 2001; Parreñas 2001a, b; Ehrenreich and Hochschild 2003; Parella 2003; Reynolds and Zontini 2006).

The 'new maid issue' can be explained by the changed need for child, health, and elderly care in private households, mainly in rich countries, caused by changes in the family structure, the increasing workforce participation of women, the growing need for assistance and nursing of the elderly, as well as the ongoing privatisation of the public care systems (Geissler 2002). To cope with and meet this demand, families increasingly resort to support outside of the family or delegate care to paid labour. Here, household workers with a migration background play an important role as they, unlike native workers in many cases, are more prepared to accept the poorly paid, insecure jobs, and precarious working conditions that characterise this sector.

Other studies have underscored ways in which transnational families are able to maintain multi-layered relationships and to develop transborder forms of social support (Goulbourne and Chamberlain 2001; Herrera Lima 2001; Bryceson and Vuorela 2002; Pribilsky 2004). Overall, the research to date has mainly focused on the positive impact of transnational care practices. In doing so, it runs the risk of losing sight of their burdensome, restrictive, and negative consequences.

Wang and Lin offer a different perspective in their study of Taiwan. The feminist perspective of the study on which this chapter draws critically examines the transfer of filial responsibilities to migrant workers, and the resulting family reorganisation that takes place by hiring a stranger to implement family care work. The authors contextualise the growing need for home care workers, the current Taiwanese policies of migration, and the private-public distribution of financial and labour responsibilities against the backdrop of the traditional value of filial piety and gendered responsibility for family care that is upheld by the social policy arrangements. Consequently, the logic of the privatised market of employment is integrated into a traditional family arrangement. The authors argue that the overall effect of these new care relationships is to perpetuate forms of oppression among women, no longer framed intergenerationally within the family but redirected at the employer-employee relationship between the daughter-in-law and the foreign migrant care worker. Such conflictual relationships are further shaped by racialised notions regarding the country of origin of the care workers. The migrant workers, highly dependent on their employers, and deprived of the legal rights to organise among themselves, turn for support primarily to their peer-group relations and informal and church-related activities.

Both chapters discuss questions of continuity and transformation of families and gendered positions in the context of transnationalism. Both underscore the socially vulnerable position of the women migrants. Both indicate that the 'experiences' can only be understood as filtered by history, policy arrangements, private-public responsibilities, values of individualism vs. collective responsibility, and a focus on women. The chapters do not point to simple 'solutions' (certainly not a panacea), neither to clearly defined 'compromises' with gains and losses for the families. They highlight a much more troubling set of transnational circumstances, further complicated by the existing formal support mechanisms which often fail to respond to their needs.

In the fourth section of this volume we analyse transnational social support from a biographical perspective. Although a variety of studies inquire into the impact of transnational social support on the social actors' life situations, few have done so from a biographical point of view. This section addresses ways in which transnational social support is embedded in the actors' life courses: how the specific biography of the subjects has an impact on the forms of social support that are developed, and the biographical meaning attributed to giving and receiving social support in a transnational context.

Bender, Hollstein, Huber, and Schweppe describe the results of a case study reconstructing the relevance of transnational social support at different stages of the migration processes. Analysing narrative-generating guided interviews, they illustrate how transnational social support is strongly linked to family members and to the presence of compatriots. In this chapter transnational social support does not seem to be a question of individual coping strategies and resources. It highlights instead the question of solidarity and how it is established.

Tuider reconstructs the biography of a migrated *maquila*-worker who lives in Ciudad Juárez. Based on research of transnational motherhood, she focuses on processes of delimitation and limitation in the everyday life of women. Tuider elaborates new practices of motherhood in the biographical representations discussed in this chapter. 'Doing family' and organising motherhood in a context of transmigration are further discussed through the perspective of feminist debates.

The previous chapters point out the potential of the transnational opening of the concept of social support to confront its prominent nation-state bias. However, the notion of transnational social support in itself needs a critical analysis. Transnationalism and transnational social support—as any other theoretical notion—are based on specific understandings of social realities and might imply unintended consequences. Therefore, the last two chapters raise critical questions with regard to the concept of transnational social support and its implicit assumptions.

Chambon and Dylan start from the observation of the absence of Aboriginal peoples in transnational studies in general and in the analysis of transnational social support in particular. They argue that transnationalism is based on a specific—modern– notion of the nation-state that is different from earlier notions which are defined "by a people in ethnic language or cultural terms." From a conception of modern nation-states, Indigenous people are considered as lacking a nation status. The authors consider that this might be part of the reason why transboundary movements across the borders of First Nations communities into the dominant society or into other First Nations are not straightforwardly perceived as transnational practices. To counteract this view, Chambon and Dylan illustrate a range of transnational—historical as well as contemporary—practices of Aboriginal peoples in Canada at the local, national, and international levels which have a high relevance for the study of transnational social support.

Köngeter turns to the question of transnational knowledge building. He approaches this theme historically using the example of Alix Westerkamp's "Letters from American Settlements," which he considers as an early example of transnational knowledge building. He bases his analysis on the concept of 'travelling theory.' His chapter reveals paradoxical phenomena within the transnational production of knowledge and especially points out as one of the consequences the reinforcement of the nation as an imagined community.

We would like to thank the authors for their collaboration as well as Routledge for accepting and publishing this volume. Our gratitude goes particularly to Max Novick from Routledge who stood by us with great calm and fortitude. We also would like to thank very much the German Research Foundation (Deutsche Forschungsgemeinschaft) for the financial support of this publication. Special thanks to Manuela Popovici for her thorough copy editing, Sarah Haese for her reliable and careful formatting, and Eva Stauf for taking on the coordination of this publication.

## NOTES

1. Internationality, by contrast, describes the relations between states, in which the states present themselves as sovereign actors (according to international law) (cf. Kaelble, Kirsch, and Schmidt-Gernig 2002). From an international

perspective, the national unity of the corresponding countries remains in the foreground as a systematic reference.

## BIBLIOGRAPHY

Anderson, B. (2000) *Doing the Dirty Work: The Global Politics of Domestic Labour.* London: Zed Books.

Bryceson, D., and U. Vuorela, eds. (2002) *The Transnational Family. New European Frontiers and Global Networks.* New York: Berg.

Ehrenreich, B., and A. R. Hochschild, eds. (2003) *Global Women. Nannies, Maids, and Sex Workers in the New Economy.* New York: Henry Holt and Company.

Elias, N. (1986) *Was ist Soziologie.* Weinheim/München: Juventa.

Faist, Th. (2000a) *The Volume and Dynamics of International Migration and Transnational Social Spaces.* Oxford: Oxford University Press.

Faist, Th., ed. (2000b) *Transstaatliche Räume. Politik, Wirtschaft und Kultur in und zwischen Deutschland und der Türkei.* Bielefeld: Transcript.

Frantz, Ch., and K. Martens (2006) *Nichtregierungsorganisationen (NGOs).* Wiesbaden: VS Verlag.

Geissler, B. (2002) 'Die Dienstmädchenlücke im Haushalt. Der neue Bedarf nach Dienstleistungen und die Handlungslogik der privaten Arbeit.' In *Weltmarkt Privathaushalt. Bezahlte Hausarbeit im globalen Wandel,* edited by C. Gather, B. Geissler, and M. S. Rerrich, 10–29. Münster: Westfälisches Dampfboot.

Glick Schiller, N., ed. (1992) *Towards a Transnational Perspective on Migration: Race, Class, Ethnicity, and Nationalism Reconsidered.* New York: John Hopkins University Press.

Global Commission on International Migration (2005) *Migration in an Interconnected World. New directions for Action.* Geneva: Global Commission on International Migration.

Goetze, D. (2002) *Entwicklungssoziologie.* Weinheim/München: Juventa.

Goulbourne, H., and M. Chamberlain, eds. (2001) *Caribbean Families in the Trans-Atlantic World.* London: Caribbean.

Herrera Lima, F. (2001) 'Transnational Families: Institutions of Transnational Social Spaces.' In *New Transnational Social Spaces,* edited by L. Pries, 77–92. London: Routledge.

Hochschild, A. R. (2000) 'Global Care Chains and Emotional Surplus Value.' In *On the Edge,* edited by W. Hutton and A. Giddens, 130–46. London: Jonathan Cape.

Hofmann, J. (2006) '(Trans-)Formations of Civil Society in Global Governance Contexts—Two Case Studies on the Problem of Self-Organization.' In *Global Governance and the Role of Non-State Actors,* edited by G. F. Schuppert, 179–202. Baden-Baden: Nomos.

Homfeldt, H. G., W. Schröer, and C. Schweppe, eds. (2008) *Soziale Arbeit und Transnationalität. Herausforderungen eines spannungsreichen Bezugs.* Weinheim und München: Juventa.

Hondagneu-Sotelo, P. (2001) *Domestica. Immigrant Workers Cleaning in the Shadows of Affluence.* London u.a.: University of California Press.

Kaelble, H., M. Kirsch, and A. Schmidt-Gernig. (2002) 'Zur Entwicklung transnationaler Öffentlichkeiten und Identitäten im 20.Jahrhundert. Eine Einleitung.' In *Transnationale Öffentlichkeiten und Identitäten im 20. Jahrhundert,* edited by H. Kaelble, M. Kirsch, and A. Schmidt-Gernig, 7–33. Frankfurt a.M.: Campus.

Kern, K. (2004) 'Globale Governance durch transnationale Netzwerkorganisationen. Möglichkeiten und Grenzen zivilgesellschaftlicher Selbstorganisation.'

In *Zivilgesellschaft—national und transnational*, edited by D. Gosewinkel, 285–308. Berlin: Edition Sigma.

Laireiter, A., and K. Lettner (1993) 'Belastende Aspekte sozialer Netzwerke und sozialer Unterstützung: Ein Überblick über den Phänomenbereich und die Methodik.' In *Soziales Netzwerk und soziale Unterstützung: Konzepte, Methoden und Befunde*, edited by A. Laireiter, 101–14. Bern u.a.: Verlag Hans Huber.

Levitt, P., and S. Khagram, eds. (2007) *The Transnational Studies Reader: Intersections and Innovations*. London/New York: Routledge.

McCall, T. (2003) 'Institutional Design for Community Economic Development Models: Issues of Opportunity and Capacity.' *Community Development Journal*, 38(2): 96–108.

Negi, N. J., and R. Furman, eds. (2010) *Transnational Social Work Practice*. New York: Columbia University Press.

Nestmann, F. (2001) 'Soziale Netzwerke—Soziale Unterstützung.' In *Handbuch Sozialarbeit/Sozialpädagogik*, edited by H. U. Otto and H. Thiersch, 1684–93. Neuwied: Luchterhand.

Parella, S. (2003) 'Immigrant Women in Paid Domestic Service. The Case of Spain and Italy.' *Transfer: European Review of Labour and Research*, 9(39): 503–17.

Parreñas, R. S. (2001a) *Servants of Globalization. Women, Migration, and Domestic Work*. Stanford: Stanford University Press.

Parreñas, R. S. (2001b) 'Mothering from a Distance: Emotions, Gender and Inter-Generational relations in Filipino Transnational Families.' *Feminist Studies*, 27(2): 361–90.

Pierce, G. R., B. R. Sarason, and I. G. Sarason, eds. (1996) *Handbook of Social Support and the Family*. New York: International Universities Press.

Pribilsky, J. (2004) '"Aprendemos a vivir': Conjugal Relations, Co-Parenting, and Family Life among Ecuadorian Transnational Migrants in New York City and the Ecuadorian Andes.' *Global Networks*, 4(3): 313–34.

Pries, L., ed. (2001) *New Transnational Social Spaces*. London/New York: Routledge.

Pries, L. (2002) 'Transnationalisierung der sozialen Welt?' *Berliner Journal für Soziologie*, 11(2): 263–72.

Pries, L. (2010) *Transnationalisierung. Theorie end Empirie grenzüberschreitender Vergesellschaft*. Wiesbaden: VS Verlag.

Reynolds, T., and E. Zontini (2006) *A Comparative Study of Care and Provision Across Caribbean and Italian Transnational Families*. London: South Bank University.

Sherraden, M., and W. Ninacs, eds. (1998) *Community Economic Development and Social Work*. New York: Routledge.

Vertovec, S. (2009) *Transnationalism (Key Ideas)*. London: Routledge.

Westwood, S., and A. Phizacklea (2000) *Transnationalism and the Politics of Belonging*. London: Taylor & Francis Ltd.

# Part I

# Transnational Social Policy

# 2 Transnational Social Policy and Migration

*Ernie Lightman*

## INTRODUCTION

Although transnational migrations have been occurring as long as there have been national borders to cross, only recently has the process become an area of interest for social work. Social work, as a profession, has long been linked with the processes and outcomes of immigration, ranging from work in early settlement houses to contemporary refugee claimants. As large numbers of migrants cross borders, perhaps thousands of miles away from their homes, arriving without obvious sources of support and facing discrimination in their daily lives, it has been the task of social work to help address their needs and concerns.

Many of these new arrivals were what we today would label as 'transnational' migrants, coming and going, perhaps through multiple countries, maintaining links of varying intensities with the places through which they transit as well as with their home countries—including in some cases an explicit intent to return, which may or may not be eventually actualised (Levitt and Jaworsky 2007; Vertovec 2009).

It is only relatively recently that social work has begun to draw distinctions between transnational migrants and the more classic one-way migration whereby people leave country A for country B, in search of economic advancement and/or greater personal freedom and security. Yet the complexities posed by the multiple and overlapping migration patterns and associated loyalties that face transnational migrants were not recognised in earlier times. Migrants—immigrants—were seen as a relatively homogenous category of clients for whom the country of receipt, the country where they likely first engaged with social work, was the primary or often the sole focus. Services were to be delivered to those in need (including immigrants) and, according to more recent practice, were to be provided in a culturally sensitive manner (Al-Ali and Koser 2002; Foner 1997).

In recent years, social workers have begun to recognise that for many, migration is not a simple one-way movement, and that linkages with other countries remain a matter of importance for many new migrants. Hence, we witness the arrival of 'transnationalism' as new terminology in the practice lexicon (Midgley 2001). Yet, the practice questions remain broadly unaltered: Care is to be provided, but whose responsibility is this? What is the role of the sending society? Of the receiving society? Of other places through which migrants may have passed and sojourned?

Most of the social work focus has lain with the direct provision of services, at the individual or micro level. This suggests a need for a further dimension to the study of transnational social work that would highlight transnational social policy. It is the purpose of this chapter to introduce transnational social policy as a formal component in the general discussions of transnationalism in social work. In so doing we limit our focus to the area of transmigration and do not consider other dimensions of transnational social policy.

Before proceeding to a formal definition of transnational social policy, it may be useful to consider a brief example, to illustrate the kinds of concerns that the concept will add to practice and understanding: Migrants, whether transnational or not, have always sent remittances to families that they left behind. From a classic social work perspective, this is a relevant concern in the receiving countries in that it adversely affects the ability of new arrivals to integrate, accumulate savings, and raise their standards of living. In the sending countries, families become dependent on these remittances, experiencing high vulnerability should there be any interruptions in the flow of currency. Each of these analyses is limited to the family level and each occurs independently of the other. From a transnational perspective, whereby the impacts on sending and receiving countries will be considered in tandem and from a policy perspective, entirely new questions arise. For example, the receipt of transnational cash flows in certain countries (such as the Philippines or Mexico) becomes an important component of national income, a large budget line for governments (Basok 2003; Goldring 2000; Guarnizo 2003; Smith 2000). Issues of concern may include the effect of these flows on the social and economic structures of the societies that rely on remittances; the gap between those who receive money from abroad and those who do not, resulting in new socio-economic classes of precariously affluent residents, dependent on relatives abroad; issues of taxation and redistribution of income and opportunities resulting from these flows; the ability of local governments to abdicate (or privatise) their roles in pursuing social justice, health, or education, and relying instead on private remittances from abroad; and the ability to cope should the flows be interrupted or reduced or inadequate to deal with unanticipated domestic crises. What happens in countries such as those in the Caribbean when their earlier role as purveyor of nannies and caregivers to Canada is superseded by new and more desirable workers from East Asia: what are the impacts on social stability, on gross domestic product and balance of payments, or on domestic unemployment levels?

Comparable concerns arise in the host countries that receive the transnational migrants (Jackson, Crang, and Dwyer 2004; Reitz 2009): What are the impacts on collective well-being when large amounts of money are sent abroad in remittances, leaving the senders potentially dependent on the state? Whose responsibility is it to care for these 'voluntarily poor' immigrants? What is the effect on local wage rates and employment levels when transnational migrants willingly work for sub-market wages, because the levels are still far above anything available in their home countries and these wages are typically paid in cash, thereby removing the money from the tax system? The combined effect in some cases is to render these transnational migrants at greater risk of financial dependency on the state, while removing their incomes from scrutiny of the local tax regimes.

We might also note that the questions just posed lie at the heart of transnational social policy, and must be addressed whether the migrants are truly transnationals or not. That is, the *process* (which we explore in this chapter) is one of transnationalism regardless of whether or not all/most/some of the migrants themselves would be considered transnationals.


## DEFINITIONS OF TRANSNATIONAL SOCIAL POLICY

In approaching a definition of transnational social policy, it is important to not be limited by the classic (particularly American) approach of social work that views policy as the outcome or consequence of decisions made at the family level. Instead, we view policy as the broad context or framework which influences and within which micro-level family decisions are made.

There are two ways to approach a definition of transnational social policy: each builds on existing definitions of social policy, while adding in a new dimension to incorporate transnationalism.

Firstly, a simple straightforward definition would refer to those initiatives, programmes, and services *intended to meet the needs of transnational migrants*. The emphasis here on the meeting of needs is directly in line with the traditional concerns of direct practice in social work and follows from early, mostly U.S.-focused definitions of social policy as meeting the needs of vulnerable members of the community (Gil 1976). Such an approach views transnational migrants as simply a subset of the broader society.

A more sophisticated definition builds on the early work of Richard Titmuss (1974), as extended by Lightman (2003). This approach looks at the two words *social* and *policy*, interpreting the meaning of each. The word *policy* implies *choice*: we have policies over those issues where we have some control and therefore are in a position to make choices; we do not have policies—and therefore do not exercise choices—over those issues where we have no control. We have no policy over whether the sun will shine tomorrow because we have no control over this; but we do have policies—we exercise choices—over what we will do if the sun does shine. The word *social* refers to groups or collectives, as distinct from individuals. One individual, in isolation, does not constitute a group (or a *society*); two or more individuals interacting in some way comprise a *social* unit.

Thus, *social policy* (taking the two words together) refers to choices and decisions that affect groups of people, as distinct from decision-making that affects only individuals (Lightman 2003). By extension, transnational social policy can be viewed as *those* choices and decisions *that affect transnational migrants and the processes of transnational migration*. Note that this definition includes both the people involved as migrants and also the processes of migration that they experience: in this discussion we focus primarily on the processes themselves which would qualify as 'transnational' whether or not the migrants are transnationals.

The choices and decisions that influence social policy can take diverse forms: They can be made by any groups in society, including residents, governments, and/or the voluntary sector; they can be focused on and/or funded by any of the societies with which the migrants—transnational or not—come into contact; the choices and decisions can be formal (legislated) or informal (ground-level practices); they can be explicit or merely implied, in the latter case leaving much discretion to individual administrators at every level, to social workers, to police, etc.; the choices can be occasional or continuing, major or minor, 'fair' or 'unfair.'

The rhetoric and the reality can be similar or widely divergent: For example, borders can be formally open, but migrants may experience harassment once they arrive; or borders may be formally closed to certain groups but in practice there is substantial movement across of excluded people and goods. As well, the formal right to work for migrants and the actual employment practices they experience may bear little relation to one another. Formal entitlement to or disqualification from benefits for migrants may be encoded and formalised, or may be dependent on the moods and practices of field-level officials; and even if rules are formalised there always remains a role for discretion and ground-level interpretation.

The second definition of transnational social policy is broader than the first, in that it does not begin with the needs of individuals and families and goes beyond the provision of services to transnational migrants; with its focus of choices and decisions as a transnational process, it readily incorporates alternative approaches to the meeting of needs and the implicit notion of limited resources. (To choose means that we opt for A at the expense of B, because we cannot do both). Thus this definition takes us to a higher level of analysis than that embedded in a simple meeting of needs, suggesting more aggregate questions of collective choices and priorities.

*Transnational social policy* is thus a macro-level component of transnational social support. It *influences* or *determines* the forms of micro-level transnational social support through decisions at the legislative, administrative, and local programmatic level; and it also *follows from* or *responds to* prior legislative, administrative, and programmatic decisions about the nature and forms of transnational social support.

Perhaps the notion of social policy is inherently a transnational concept: The definition of *social* in *social policy* (earlier) refers to societies, communities, collectives, groups (Lightman 2003, following Titmuss 1974). It makes no explicit reference to the nation-state or to national boundaries which are prerequisite for transnationalism. Thus, the generic definition of social policy previously developed in the literature already incorporates or accommodates a transnational dimension; or, in other words, social policy, by its very definition, is not limited to the boundaries or structures of the nation-state (although it was always developed within a nation-state). Perhaps, then, our existing definitions are sufficient and we need not extend them further.

At the same time, the notion of a *border* appears crucial to any understanding of transnational social policy. Without a border, one cannot cross from country to country and hence, almost by definition, there can be no transnational migration. Crossing a border makes one a *visitor*, an *immigrant*, or an *alien*, depending on the particular circumstances, and regardless of whether the border was crossed legally or illegally, temporarily or permanently, with or without papers. Each of the three terms conveys a distinct status to those crossing and carries with it certain specific legal implications (Mahler 2001).

Consider, for example, a worker from Newfoundland who travels to Alberta in search of employment. This person maintains ongoing contact with home, returns frequently to visit, may send cash remittances on a regular basis, and, when laid off, may well return home permanently. This person fulfills all the criteria for a transnational migrant except that s/he does not cross a border. As a Canadian citizen, s/he has certain rights and privileges wherever s/he travels in the country. The unemployment insurance programme, for example, is national in scope (though benefit levels do vary regionally).

Compare this person to the worker from Latin America, who travels roughly the same distance, also to work in the tar sands of Alberta. S/he also maintains regular contact with home, undoubtedly sends cash remittances, and may (or may not) visit or return home when laid off. If this person is in Canada with proper papers, s/he has certain rights which may well be less than those that accrue to citizens or permanent residents; if this person comes without documentation, s/he has few rights at all and is vulnerable to ongoing exploitation.

The only difference between these two cases is that one stays within a formal national border, while the other crosses a border or two. While the latter is labelled a *transnational migrant,* the former might be called an *intranational migrant* (within a single nation-state). Though their employment situations may be identical, their need for social support, whether formal or informal, is likely to differ, and their inclusion in state social policies will also diverge. As a result, their reliance on social supports from the voluntary sector will also be different. Yet, in reality, the only factor distinguishing their situation is that one of them crosses a formal legal border while the other does not. One may be in need of transnational social support (which s/he may or may not receive) while the other will have access to more traditional mainstream social services (Bernhard, Landolt, and Goldring 2005; Vertovec 2009).

## THE CONTEXT OF TRANSNATIONAL SOCIAL POLICY

The academic literature on transnational social policy first becomes visible in the early 1990s. There is some earlier material that deals with the phenomenon, though it does not appear to use the label as such (Levitt and Jaworsky 2007; Vertovec 2009).

However, the practice of transnationalism is much older. Prior to World War I, there were no widespread guarded borders within either Europe or North America: people were relatively free to travel from place to place, from country to country. Typically they were seeking something such as a higher income or personal freedom, or they were fleeing from something, usually oppression of some sort. These voyagers usually maintained links with their original places and some returned regularly, particularly if the geographic distances were not great. Because the notion of the nation-state with clearly defined borders was relatively undeveloped at this time, so too the concept of transnationalism (which entails crossing clearly defined borders) was little understood or even recognised. Social supports to these transnational migrants were provided only through the voluntary sector—often cultural, ethnic, or faith communities—which were also not bound by national borders.

The first major state role in providing social services emerged in the English-speaking world only after World War II. The Keynes-Beveridge welfare state, as it was known, was based on the macroeconomics of Keynes and the social policy of Beveridge. This model was inherently a project of the nation-state: Keynes's original mathematical models were limited to a closed economy, with neither exports nor imports, an approach that created difficulties as international trade became ever more prominent. For example, the exogenously induced inflation which most countries experienced after the dramatic rise in world oil prices in the 1970s could not be addressed through traditional Keynesian approaches of reducing aggregate demand. It was not until years after Keynes completed his work that other economists expanded the original models beyond the nation-state focus, and even today Keynesianism is limited in its ability to undertake international analyses (Lightman 2003).

Likewise, in most cases, the new post-war welfare states had a national focus. Typically this was reflected through eligibility criteria that limited entitlement to those meeting them. In some cases, formal citizenship was required (as with voting in national elections); in other cases, a minimum period of legal residence was necessary (as with Canada's non-contributory Old Age Security pensions); at times legal residence or presence was sufficient (as with school enrolment in some jurisdictions). Occasionally, and unusually, there were no further requirements for eligibility beyond physical presence in a jurisdiction. For many years after its introduction in 1949, Britain's National Health Service (NHS) was available on equal terms to all persons physically present in the country, including new arrivals, regardless of legal status. This approach was based on a philosophical value system that talked of community and rejected distinctions based on legal status. By the 1970s, however, a strong sense of abuse—people arriving in Britain solely to secure needed and typically expensive medical care without charge—led to more explicit residency requirements in the NHS (Glennerster 2000, 2003). To the extent these benefits were based on residence rather than citizenship, transnational migrants had little difficulty securing coverage, often on the same terms as native-born residents; but over time, formal legal status in the country has become more important, often leaving transnational migrants—particularly transients—without entitlements or benefits. This has placed greater onus on the voluntary sector to fill in the gaps resulting from state withdrawal as service provider.

More recently, the nation-state in Europe has given way to the European Union, but this evolution does not alter our analysis. The notion of 'borders' or 'boundaries' to identify those eligible for support remains the same, though the specific boundaries have expanded outward to encompass many or all the countries that comprise the EU (Ginsburg 2001).

Also in recent years, the forces of globalisation have threatened the traditional welfare state. *Globalisation* (in this context, using U.S. definitions) implies the reduction or elimination of national boundaries and their replacement by the impersonal rules of the economic market. National governments become subservient to international economic forces, limited in their ability to offset domestically the outcomes of international economic decision-making (Vertovec 2004; Wimmer and Glick Schiller 2003). This results in the consequent inability of the nation-state to introduce or maintain social welfare measures for either domestic or migrant, permanent or temporary populations for at least two reasons. Firstly, when national social priorities conflict with the law of contract, the latter typically takes precedence. For example, occupational health and safety regulations must often give way to contrary dictates in commercial contracts. Secondly, because globalisation renders capital highly mobile, investment flows to places where the return/profit is greatest: these will often be settings in which both taxes and wages are low, leaving no room for social welfare measures. High wage–high tax countries are at risk of being left on the sidelines as investment and jobs flow to the more compliant alternatives. At the same time, the reduced importance of borders resulting from globalisation has led to increased migration, including transnational migration, resulting in greater need for transnational social support (Levitt and Glick

Schiller 2004). Yet, for the reasons just indicated, governments have been unwilling or incapable of providing this.

The weakening of the forces of globalisation in recent years has been accompanied by the re-emergence of the nation-state (or, in some case, the theocratic state). Former British Prime Minister Gordon Brown referred to the processes of 'de-globalisation' in the context of the global financial melt-down of 2009 ('Deglobalization a new threat to the world, Brown warns' 2009). In principle, this should make migration more difficult and should be associated with reduced flows of people from country to country. In practice, however, this has not occurred. The xenophobia associated with the new nation-states has made minority and other vulnerable groups ever more desperate to leave; and the widening economic gaps between the rich and poor countries have likewise increased incentives to migration. If legal population flows are suppressed, the drive to migrate will manifest itself illegally, as in the boatloads of immigrants without papers that arrive on Canada's west coast from time to time. In Europe, the Roma populations can be evicted from France in the name of the new nation-state parochialism, but no one seriously believes the underlying migration of peoples from east to west in Europe will cease or even diminish substantially. Immigrants without papers, almost by definition, have reduced formal social protections—in practice, even if not in principle—and thus their social needs are likely to remain unaddressed by the state. Once again, even greater responsibilities will fall into the ever-shrinking laps of the voluntary sector. The meeting of social needs is dramatically shifting from the state to the private sector (which includes of course the entire voluntary sector) and transnational migrants are among those affected by these changes.

## THE PROCESSES AND OUTCOMES OF TRANSNATIONAL SOCIAL POLICY

In general terms, transnational social policy is associated with transnational population flows (though the causality can be in either direction). There has always been both a 'push' and a 'pull' to the migration: The 'pull' is usually associated with the pursuit of a better life and economic opportunities, as in 'the streets of New York are paved with gold.' The 'push' is often associated with flight from oppression or persecution, as people run from wars, genocides, and economic crises; however, 'push' can also be a conscious developmental strategy, as in the Philippines, where people are trained to be exported as nannies and caregivers abroad. Transnational migration is distinguished from traditional migration in that it is not solely a one-way movement from A to B; rather it is associated with multiple dimensions of interaction among different countries as mobile individuals maintain and sever links of various sorts with the home country, and potentially several transit and receiving countries. The cause and nature of the population movements clearly influence the nature of the need for transnational social services, in both sending and receiving countries (Faist 2000; Wayland 2006).

- The need for transnational social policies is based on four general considerations. How these manifest themselves and how they interact will determine whether there will be transnational linkages and what their strength and resilience will be. They refer both to context and individuals, thus operating at both the macro and the micro levels. The policies and practices, both formal and informal, in the sending or initial countries: Do they have programmes or initiatives in place to encourage or facilitate transnational linkages? Do they erect barriers? Are they indifferent? Some countries (such as Ireland or Iceland) actively promote transnational linkages, both through government missions abroad and through support of the voluntary sector. St Patrick's Day celebrations in many countries, the symbolism of the shamrock and the leprechaun, even Guinness beer, all promote a positive image abroad for the Irish nation-state while also helping migrants maintain their transnational linkages with the home country. Other countries such as North Korea make such links difficult to maintain and actively discourage the 'to and fro' flows of transnationalism.
- The policies and practices, both formal and informal, in the receiving countries (noting there may be multiple transit and receiving countries as transnational migrants represent ongoing population movements): Do the receiving countries have programmes or initiatives in place to encourage or facilitate transnational linkages? Do they erect barriers? Are they indifferent? Some practices can evolve without a formal governmental role: Ong and Nonini (1997), for example, identified Chinese transnationalism across Southeast Asia as responsible for the spread of Confucian values in the development of social policy in that region (Ong and Nonini 1997).
- The personal priorities and preferences of transnational migrants: Some individuals value these transnational links highly and work to maintain them, while others, often for personal reasons, have no particular interest in transnationalism.
- The technical ease or difficulty for transnational migrants to maintain links with home countries: Although telecommunications and transportation have become dramatically cheaper in recent years, for a long time cost considerations made transnationalism harder to maintain in some places. Even today, it is still difficult to support such links to certain countries and regions.

Traditional social policy (Lightman 2003) is based on answers to a limited number of broad questions: with modification, these same questions help in understanding the processes of transnational social policy. Perhaps the most central of these questions asks whose responsibility it is to meet needs, both individual and collective. Is the role assigned to individuals (as in the traditional economic market) or to the collective/group/community/society? And if the latter is involved, does this entail action by government or by the voluntary/non-governmental sector (or both, in varying combinations)?

In focusing on transnational social policy, we add a new dimension to these questions: Given that there are at least two distinct societies—one sending and one receiving—and possibly many more, which of the multiple societies holds responsibility for the meeting of these needs for transnational migrants? Which government(s) and which voluntary agency/ies? And, given that there are multiple flows back and forth—commodities, money, communications, travel, and other linkages—how are the key questions to be answered for each of these factors individually?

More specifically, does the original initiating society have obligations towards those who migrate, either temporarily or permanently? For example, Canada's Old Age Security (OAS), a universal non-contributory taxable monthly payment to those 65 and older who meet certain residency (not citizenship) requirements is receivable worldwide, through direct bank transfer in some cases; on the other hand, the Guaranteed Income Supplement (GIS), a means-tested supplement to low-income seniors, is payable only in Canada to current Canadian residents. From this we infer that Canada holds an obligation to those seniors who spend at least twenty years of their adult lives in the country but this does not extend to meet the low-income needs of those who choose to sojourn or reside abroad.

Does the receiving society/ies have any obligation to meet the needs of those arriving at its borders, whether temporarily or permanently? We noted earlier the example of Britain's National Health Service (NHS), originally available on equal terms to all those physically present in the country, regardless of legal status, but subsequently tightened in the face of significant system 'abuse.' More recently (*Toronto Star* 9 March 2009), the province of Quebec has identified a problem with 'maternity tourism,' whereby women, often from French-speaking countries, arrive in Quebec in the late stages of pregnancy, give birth (thereby securing citizenship for the child), and leave the country without paying the hospital and medical bills.

Because the welfare state is based on the concept of the nation-state, the integration of new residents, whether transnational migrants or new permanent residents, has always been problematic. There is a dichotomy, by which one either qualifies for social benefits, or one does not, and the criteria by which one becomes eligible vary from programme to programme, from jurisdiction to jurisdiction. Often there is a waiting period: new residents to Ontario, for example, face a 90-day period before they become eligible for health care (Medicare) benefits. When parents are in Canada without documentation, the rights of their children to attend school are often murky; Old Age Security (OAS) requires twenty years' residence in Canada (after age eighteen) in order to qualify for full payment, while the benefits are pro-rated for lesser periods of time. Both transnational, temporary migrants and permanent new immigrants would face these same barriers to accessing benefits (Stewart et al. 2006) assuming the former are in the country with correct papers; those without papers have few rights.

Over the years, a number of creative initiatives have been developed to meet the needs of immigrants without fundamentally challenging the nation-state focus of the welfare state. For example, many schools now pursue "Don't ask; don't tell" policies with respect to the schooling of children: they do not inquire into the residence status of parents and it is assumed parents will not volunteer this information. In this way, the children can get access to the full school system. In addition, there has been considerable growth in the number of NGOs that attempt to meet needs resulting from these gaps in coverage and, at the same time, advocate for changes in the regulatory frameworks. The goal, in most cases, is to work towards a system of social services in which eligibility is based on need rather than legal status or time in the country. While these initiatives do not specifically target transnational migrants—and in fact are often directed more towards refugee claimants, whether transnational or not—the effect is to extend service coverage to all those in need, regardless of status.

But transnationalism has added new dimensions to these debates over entitlement. At times, transnational migrants will claim to be permanent residents/immigrants (or will pretend) in order to claim benefits, e.g., for many years (and perhaps still today, though to a lesser extent), American residents close to the Canadian border would pretend to be transnationals, living in Canada enough days to qualify for health coverage. As a result, qualification requirements for health benefits have been tightened severely in recent years to close this expensive 'loophole' in the system. In other cases, people will not disclose absences abroad: continuing coverage under Medicare requires physical presence in Ontario for 186 days a year; the Guaranteed Income Supplement for low-income seniors is available only to those permanently resident in Canada. Once again formerly loose eligibility determination has been tightened in recent years.

The legal framework can facilitate or impede access to benefits for transnational migrants, by rigour of enforcement (as noted earlier) and through the actual content of the laws themselves: for example, the law can specify a formal finite length of time one can be in Canada under certain programmes, and when this time is up, the visitor must then either leave the country or remain without papers. The more the laws and their enforcement are framed to serve a gatekeeper function—to deny and exclude from entitlement—clearly the more difficult it becomes for transnationals to receive needed services. The legal framework can also facilitate or impede the maintenance of transnational linkages, which can at times serve as a substitute for the receipt of local services. The law can attempt to distinguish permanent immigrants from transnational migrants to provide benefits for the former but not the latter, but this is hard to do, as the two categories are not mutually exclusive: *a claimant can simultaneously be a permanent immigrant (a legal status) and a transnational migrant (a behavioural condition).*

Both the initiating and the receiving societies can develop initiatives to protect the interests of transnational migrants, or they can decline to do so. The sending societies can permit people to carry benefits wherever they may choose to reside, as occurs, for example, with Canada's Old Age Security payments. They can more formally advocate with receiving societies to protect the interests and needs of migrants through the introduction of anti-discrimination legislation or practices: for example, those countries that send caregivers or labourers abroad will attempt (usually unsuccessfully) to protect their nationals against undue personal abuse or exploitation through unsafe working practices. In some cases, sending countries can fund or support agencies or NGOs in the receiving societies that include in their mandates the interests of transnational migrants.

The receiving societies, for their part, can introduce legal protections for transnational migrants through anti-discrimination legislation that is effectively enforced. They may also overlook extra-legal practices by transnational migrants that serve as a form of self-help to meet needs that are otherwise unaddressed. And they can also fund or support new or existing NGOs that (re)define their mandates to include services to transnational migrants.

In all these cases, voluntary agencies or NGOs can emerge to address the gaps in service provision for transnational migrants. These agencies may be partially funded by governments, either in the service-providing countries or elsewhere, or they may be totally independent of governments that choose to not intervene in the provision of services. Existing NGOs can expand their mandates to include transnationals, or new, special purpose NGOs can emerge, but in all cases their funding is likely to be tenuous, as will their ability to fulfill mandates (Cooley and Ron 2002; Jordan and Van Tuijl 2000).

To summarise this section, we can see that transnational migrants, particularly if they are present in substantial numbers, may alter the functions of the state in response to new and emerging needs that are not addressed elsewhere. The roles, functions, and expectations placed on the state may change dramatically. The state can respond by expanding its role, either directly or indirectly through supporting voluntary agencies/NGOs, thereby working towards the social inclusion of all those present in the society; or, alternatively, the state may choose to restrict its role to prevent meeting the needs of new transnational residents, thereby impeding social inclusion either actively (through new restrictive laws and regulations) or passively (by ignoring new problems). In this latter case even greater responsibility is placed on voluntary agencies/NGOs who will likely face increased demands for service from a shrinking fiscal base (Hirschman, Dewind, and Kasinitz 1999; Glick Schiller and Fouron 2001).

The *outcomes* of transnational social policy, as might be expected, relate directly to, and follow from, the processes. Hence, the outcomes will vary, dependent on the same four considerations that influence the processes:

- The conditions and attitudes in the receiving society/ies
- The conditions and attitudes in the sending society/ies
- The personal attitudes, preferences, and desires of the transnational migrants
- The technical ease or difficulty to maintain transnational links

Transnational migrants can assume a range of statuses in any or all of the societies in which they sojourn: they can be marginalised and second-class, fully integrated, or anything in between. The most extreme marginal status suggests no real sense of inclusion or integration in any of the societies through which they may pass, along with only tenuous links to the initiating society/ies. "They don't belong here and they don't belong there." This condition may result from a failure or inability of transnational social policy (both government and NGO) in any/all the affected societies to address the social and economic gaps that lead to exclusion; combined with this at the micro level, individuals may not make sufficient efforts to address their own needs (Heisler 2001).

At the other extreme, transnational migrants may be fully integrated into all of the societies with which they interact. They can move back and forth, with comfort and ease. "They belong both here and there." This fluidity of movement may occur with or without the active intervention of the affected governments and NGOs (DeMars 2005; Hondagneu-Sotelo and Avila 1997).

Finally, transnational migrants can be placed anywhere between these polar cases, or they can shift into and out of the polar cases. Where individuals and groups of transnational migrants will be found on a scale of integration/exclusion will vary with time, space, distance, context, and personal preferences and characteristics.

## FINAL THOUGHTS

This chapter has attempted to combine the existing literatures on transnationalism and on social policy to present a first look at transnational social policy and migration. In doing this, we have extended the ideas of mainstream social policy through the inclusion of a new dimension of transnationalism. The outcomes are not the same, for the addition of a new variable to the equation inevitably alters the calculus and the results. Nevertheless, we have begun to explore transnational social policy through the formulation of new questions and approaches in ways that may be helpful to other researchers.

These preliminary thoughts have not addressed a number of important questions that may serve as a conclusion to this chapter.

Firstly it is crucial to appreciate that transnational social policy does not necessarily promote positive outcomes for recipients. The original definition of social policy, which refers to 'choices' and 'options,' is consciously silent on the content or outcomes of those choices. Thus, traditional social policy can serve for good (inclusion) or bad (exclusion). Modifying the definition to encompass a transnational dimension does nothing to alter this fundamental silence. While much of this chapter has focused on how transnational social policy can serve to meet the needs of transnational migrants, the same social policy can equally serve to deny entitlements and restrict eligibility. It is only through the introduction of an exogenous value system that transnational social policy acquires either a positive or a negative vector.

Secondly, this chapter has not addressed the central role played by economic class. Not all transnational migrants are the same, and their needs differ dramatically dependent on who they are, where they come from, and what their personal, private resource packages are. Much of the literature on transnationalism refers to poor and marginalised populations who cross borders to escape economic deprivation and/or persecution. We think, immediately, of those moving from eastern Europe and Turkey to western Europe, or from the Caribbean islands, Mexico, and Central America to the United States and Canada. In all these cases, upward economic mobility is a central (though not always exclusive) motivator for movement. These transnational migrants tend to live on the margins of the receiving societies, working at precarious employment, and subject to various forms of exclusion and discrimination. If they do not hold proper documentation, their situations are even more vulnerable. That these populations need social services and supportive social policies—whether traditional nationally bounded or transnational—is rather evident (Massey, Goldring, and Durand 1994; Rouse 1992).

However, there also exists the transnational movement of middle- and upper-class migrants, who have personal social capital and considerable resources (Granovetter 1973; Vertovec 2009; Wong 2004). There are many Americans living and working in Canada who may well identify as transnationals, but who clearly do not need targeted social services and supports. Often they bring their American values promoting individualism and primacy of the private market, a process that has a deleterious effect on the maintenance of Canada's own social policies and programmes. Many of these temporary migrants live on the upper margins of Canada's economic structure, receiving particular supports (such as foreign living allowances) from the United States while also benefiting from (and simultaneously criticising) Canada's own social systems such as public health care.

Class is important. And while we may properly focus on poor and vulnerable transnational migrants as those in greatest need of our collective attention, it is also important to remember that not all transnational migrants in all countries are in need of specific added supports and concerns. Those from wealthy countries and communities are well able to look after their own interests.

We may close with a final word on the meaning of transnational immigration to Canada. Canada's traditional 'openness' to immigration—including transnational migrants—is typically associated with little or no pressure to 'become Canadian' (whatever that phrase may mean). This is often juxtaposed to the United States notion of the 'melting pot' with its implied (or perhaps more explicit) pressure to 'become American.' The difference in approach of the two countries has been attributed to various causes: the greater sense of nationalism, parochialism, and perhaps even xenophobia in the U.S. today is undoubtedly evident, but even historically the U.S. has always been focused on nation-building to a greater extent than Canada. As well, Canada receives greater numbers of immigrants relative to total population, including in recent years, and so there will be closer and more ongoing links to home countries abroad (Bumsted 2001; Lipset 1992; Reitz and Somerville 2004). This encourages greater transnational interest and hence the need for transnational services and social policies.

The implication is that there will be greater interest in, and need for, transnational social policy in Canada than in the United States. Offsetting this of course is the greater number of immigrants to the U.S. who lack documentation and hence are more socially vulnerable and at risk of discrimination and deportation.

Some have challenged the very distinction between America's 'melting pot' and Canada's lesser pressure to induce social integration (Reitz and Breton 1994). This is not the place to explore that challenge, but the distinction between the two images of the societies does remain a powerful force in creating a Canadian identity, regardless of reality on the ground.

## BIBLIOGRAPHY

Al-Ali, N., and K. Koser, eds. (2002) *New Approaches to Migration? Transnational Communities and the Transformation of Home*. New York: Routledge.

Basok, T. (2003) 'Mexican Seasonal Migration to Canada and Development: A Community-Based Comparison.' *International Migration*, 41(2): 3–26.

Bernhard, J. K., P. Landolt, and L. Goldring (2005) 'Transnational, Multi-Local Motherhood: Experiences of Separation and Reunification among Latin American Families in Canada'. University of Toronto, Joint Centre of Excellence for Research on Immigration and Settlement (CERIS), CERIS Working Paper No. 40.

Bumsted, J. (2001) 'Visions of Canada: A Brief History of Writing on the Canadian Character and the Canadian Identity.' In *A Passion for Identity: Canadian Studies for the 21st Century*, edited by D. Tara and B. Rasporich, 17–35. Toronto: Nelson College Indigenous.

Cooley, A., and J. Ron (2002) 'The NGO Scramble: Organizational Insecurity and the Political Economy of Transnational Action.' *International Security*, 27(1): 5–39.

'Deglobalization a New Threat to the World, Brown Warns.' (2009, January 20). Agence France Press. http://www.abs-cbnnews.com/world/01/19/09/de-globalization-new-threat-world-brown-warns

DeMars, W. E. (2005) *NGOs and Transnational Networks: Wild Cards in World Politics*. London: Pluto Press.

Faist, T. (2000) 'Transnationalization in International Migration: Implications for the Study of Citizenship and Culture.' *Ethnic and Racial Studies*, 22(2): 189–222.

Foner, N. (1997) 'What's New about Transnationalism? New York Immigrants Today and at the Turn of the Century.' *Diaspora*, 6(3): 355–75.

Gil, D. (1976) *The Challenge of Social Equality*. Cambridge, MA: Schenkman.

Ginsburg, N. (2001) 'Globalization and the Liberal Welfare States.' In *Globalization and European Welfare States: Challenges and Change*, edited by R. Sykes, B. Palier, and P. M. Prior, 173–91. Hampshire: Palgrave.

Glennerster, H. (2000) *British Social Policy since 1945*. Oxford: Blackwell Publishers Inc.

Glennerster, H. (2003) *Understanding the Finance of Welfare*. Bristol: The Policy Press.

Glick Schiller, N. and G. Fouron (2001) 'All in the Family: Gender, Transnational Migration, and the Nation-State.' *Identities*, 7(4): 539–82.

Goldring, L. (2000) 'Disaggregating Transnational Social Spaces: Gender, Place and Citizenship in Mexico-US Transnational Spaces.' In *New Transnational Social Spaces: International Migration and Transnational Companies in the Early 21st Century*, edited by L. Pries, 59–76. London: Routledge.

Granovetter, M. S. (1973) 'The Strength of Weak Ties.' *American Journal of Sociology*, 78: 1360–80.

Guarnizo, L. E. (2003) 'The Economics of Transnational Living.' *International Migration Review*, 37(3): 666–99.

Heisler, M. O. (2001) 'Now and Then, Here and There: Migration and the Transformation of Identities, Borders and Orders.' In *Identities, Borders, Orders*, edited by M. Albert, D. Jacobson, and Y. Lapid, 225–47. Minneapolis: University of Minnesota Press.

Hirschman, C., J. Dewind, and P. Kasinitz, eds. (1999) *The Handbook of International Migration*. New York: Russel Sage Foundation.

Hondagneu-Sotelo, P., and E. Avila (1997) '"I'm Here, but I'm There.' The Meanings of Latina Transnational Motherhood.' *Gender and Society*, 11(5): 548–71.

Jackson, P., P. Crang, and D. Dwyer, eds. (2004) *Transnational Spaces*. London: Routledge.

Jordan, L., and P. Van Tuijl (2000) 'Political Responsibility in Transnational NGO Advocacy.' *World Development*, 28(12): 2051–65.

Levitt, P., and N. Glick Schiller (2004) 'Conceptualizing Simultaneity: A Transnational Social Field Perspective on Society.' *International Migration Review*, 38(3): 1002–39.

Levitt, P., and B. N. Jaworsky (2007) 'Transnational Migration Studies: Past Developments and Future Trends.' *Annual Review of Sociology*, 33: 129–56.

Lightman, E. (2003) *Social Policy in Canada*. Toronto: Oxford.

Lipset, S. M. (1992) 'Canada and the United States Compared.' In *Canada*, edited by M. Watkins, 651–63. New York: Facts on File.

Mahler, S. (2001) 'Transnational Relationships: The Struggle to Communicate across Borders.' *Identities*, 7: 583–619.

Massey, D. S., L. Goldring, and J. Durand (1994) 'Continuities in Transnational Migration: An Analysis of Nineteen Mexican Communities.' *American Journal of Sociology*, 99(1): 492–533.

Midgley, J. (2001) 'Issues in International Social Work.' *Journal of Social Work*, 1(1): 21–35.

Ong, A., and D. Nonini, eds. (1997) *Ungrounded Empires*. London: Routledge.

Reitz, J. G. (2009) 'Assessing Multiculturalism as a Behavioural Theory.' In *Multiculturalism and Social Cohesion: Potentials and Challenges of Diversity*, edited by J. G. Reitz, R. Breton, K. K. Dion, and K. L. Dion, 1–47. New York: Springer.

Reitz, J. G., and R. Breton (1994) *The Illusion of Difference: Realities of Ethnicity in Canada and the United States*. Toronto: C. D. Howe Institute.

Reitz, J. G., and K. Somerville (2004) 'Institutional Change and Emerging Cohorts of the 'New' Immigrant Second Generation: Implications for the Integration of Racial Minorities in Canada.' *Journal of International Migration and Integration*, 5(4): 385–415.

Rouse, R. (1992) 'Making Sense of Settlement: Class Transformation, Cultural Struggle, and Transnationalism among Mexican Migrants in the United States.' *Annals of the New York Academy of Sciences*, 645: 25–52.

Smith, R. (2000) 'Comparing Local-Level Swedish and Mexican Transnational Life: An Essay in Historical Retrieval.' In *New Transnational Social Spaces: International Migration and Transnational Companies in the Early 21st Century*, edited by L. Pries, 37–58. London: Routledge.

Stewart, M. J., A. Neufeld, M. J. Harrison, D. Spitzer, K. Highes, and E. Markwarimba (2006) 'Immigrant Women Family Caregivers in Canada: Implications for Policies and Programmes in Health and Social Sectors.' *Health & Social Care in the Community*, 14(4): 329–40.

Titmuss, R. (1974) *Social Policy: An Introduction*. London: Allen and Unwin.

Toronto Star (2009). *Maternity Tourism leaves MDs footing bill*. Toronto: March 09, 2009.

Vertovec, S. (2004) 'Migrant Transnationalism and Modes of Transformation.' *International Migration Review*, 38(3): 970–1001.

Vertovec, S. (2009) *Transnationalism*. New York: Routledge.

Wayland, S. V. (2006) 'The Politics of Transnationalism: Comparative Perspectives.' In *Transnational identities and practices in Canada*, edited by V. Satzewich and L. Wong, 18–34. Vancouver: UBC Press.

Wimmer, A., and N. Glick Schiller (2003) 'Methodological Nationalism, the Social Sciences, and the Study of Migration: An Essay in Historical Epistemology.' *The International Migration Review*, 37(3): 576–610.

Wong, L. (2004) 'Taiwanese Immigrant Entrepreneurs in Canada and Transnational Social Space.' *International Migration*, 42(4): 113–52.

# 3 Social Policy in a Transnational World
## The Capability Approach, Neediness, and Social Work

*Lothar Böhnisch and Wolfgang Schröer*

"Flying blind with spectators" was the title that the futurologist Bolz (2005) chose for his attempt to forecast social developments at the start of the twenty-first century: "Modern society is moving forward as though flying blind. This is saying more than that evolution operates blindly, which is simply a statement of the obvious. Flying blind also means flying with instruments only. If you look out of the window, you can see nothing—but you can rely on the dials on the instrument panel [ . . . ] The instruments and the crew are reliable, but no one knows the destination" (9).

If we apply this to the future of social work, it could mean that under the influence of current trends, social work in western industrial societies is finding itself increasingly abandoned by the national social state, carried along by the transnational blurring of boundaries into an uncertain societal future. At the same time, in some regions it has reached an unprecedented level of professional quality and infrastructural development and feels itself strong enough not only to legitimate itself normatively and in terms of social structure, but also to prove itself transnationally in terms of its efficacy. "What works?" is now the self-confident question it asks. Or, what share of credit can social work claim for the success of a once endangered biography or of a sustainable social community?

But no sooner do we venture to consider such a perspective than the framework disappears from view, and the positional lights which should help the instruments to work become hazy on the global horizon. How will social work position itself in the future? One thing can be confidently predicted: It will be a blind flight that encounters turbulence. Social work is dependent on normative guidelines, and instrumental justification alone is not sufficient: How social work is able to develop its sphere of activity nationally and transnationally depends on the policy of social justice, on the level and clarity of the prevailing ethic of justice and responsibility, and on the equilibrium between humans and the economy. Turbulence arises not only when all this is equivocal, but when paradoxes rule the societal scene and social orientations are obscured. Bourdieu (1997) made a prediction along these lines: "More than ever before, we need to practise paradoxical thinking" (189).

When trapped in paradoxes, it is difficult to make pronouncements about the future. "Every future is the self-reflexive image of the present. And the future reconstitutes itself afresh in every present" (Bolz 2005: 17). In view of the paradoxical present, however, we are more conscious than ever that society does have a future, but that we cannot imagine what path this future might take. In the idea of 'reflexive modernisation,' which dominated the social-scientific thinking in some European countries during the transition to the twenty-first century, we were fairly confident that course corrections were possible in the confrontation between the early history of the modern age and the present time. The dynamics of globalisation seem to have negated this reflexive reference transnationally.

At the same time, we see that for the development of social work there was and is always a need for critical *Zeitdiagnosen* [diagnoses of our time] of the socio-historical developments with a socio-political dimension. Among others, Fraser (2009) follows in this tradition. In doing so, she not only uses, quite consciously, the German concept of *Zeitdiagnosen*, but also goes beyond it and remarks that the diagnoses to which, for example, the debates about a theory of social justice relate are, at present, inappropriate, or insufficiently grounded in social history. They often continue to refer to twentieth-century models of national state welfare. Many models of justice take no account of the social processes involving the dissolution of boundaries and the current field of tension between transnationality, the national state, and locality.

Naturally, a diagnosis of our time is always controversial, but it is also an essential component of critical approaches to social work. In social work, socio-political diagnoses of our time are thus currently faced with the challenge of catching up with the processes of dissolution of boundaries and of acquiring a new understanding of the dimensions of transnational, national, and local social policies: "In a world of transnational societies, the causes of—and, presumably, the solutions to—the problems of social order and security are not confined to national territories and national social structures and institutions. These problems need to be reconceptualised to account for the impact of globalisation on the capacity of the state to recreate national histories within the boundaries of national territories" (Baltodano 1999: 39).

## TRANSNATIONAL CHALLENGES TO THE NATIONAL SOCIAL STATE

At the start of the twenty-first century, in many regions the social is being refashioned more radically than anyone could have imagined twenty years ago. In globalisation, the accelerating dissolution of the boundaries of space and time has rendered the compass of the twentieth century useless by building a transnational field of magnetism in which the compass seems to swing constantly in an uncontrolled fashion. The talk of the risk society, which—in the context of 'reflexive modernisation' and in light of the incalculable consequences of modernisation—characterised the social discourse from the 1980s, has long since expanded to embrace the global risk society (cf. Beck 2007). It has given way to the fear of no longer being able to assess the new threats by means of the now obsolete crisis discourse. It seems that two worlds have arisen: a socially embedded world and a transnationally disembedded world.

In the meantime, worldwide debates about a transnational social policy are focusing on how a connection to this disembedded world can be created, in order to exert influence. It is no longer a matter of using new technological models to regulate globalisation, but of power, and of the shift of power relationships that impacts social developments on a worldwide scale. Since the 1990s, the emphasis in social policy has been placed mainly on universal rights; local and transnational communities and new 'global' and 'grassroots' movements are being invoked (cf. Morales-Gómez 1999; Jones Finer 1999).

In social work, it can be observed that such 'classical' crystallisation points of its development and socio-political reflexivity as care, commons, and citizenship are being affected in a new way by the tension between transnationality, the national state, and locality. Thus, care is currently stressing the need to look beyond the national framework, and the same thing is happening in relation to social and civil rights (citizenship) and the responsibility for public goods and the shaping of the local community (commons). The national social state ought to regulate social care arrangements (care), guarantee social rights (citizenship), bear social responsibility for public goods (commons), and must, in appropriate ways, ensure and shape the *social integration* and *development* of a society. However, currently in many countries of the West the state finds itself confronted with the dynamics of disintegration, and driven by socio-political forces into the strait-jacket of situations where social development seems scarcely possible.

For social work, this can have the effect that its perspective for integration loses any connection with society. This means that if the national social state gets into a transnationally induced integration dilemma, it must necessarily shift its integration policy away from marginal groups and into the heart of society. So if it continues to act according to the previous template of social state delegation, social work could be relegated to the functional sphere of the *administration of social marginality*. All in all, it is clear that in many places social work reflexivity must extend beyond the national social state if this new magnetic field of the rise and shaping of social problems and their transnational relationships is to be recognised.

A start has been made by means of the concept of social work as a 'human rights profession' (cf. Staub-Bernasconi 1998). We shall say no more, at this point, about how this concept relies on the optimistic view that social work can be tied more strongly to international social movements and institutions, and that it proposes a normative superstructure that is professionally non-specific, because it crosses professional boundaries and must be shared with other professions. In general, the concept is part of the mainstream of many discussions surrounding transnational social policy, which often look for a universal justification beyond the social. The national social state is no longer considered to be capable of very much. The term 'post-social state' is gaining currency in the profession.

Although the death knell might be sounded for the national social state, this does not, of course, mean that the state will not exist in the future. Social regulation and basic background security will continue to be indispensable for certain groups of persons. But the weakness of recent conceptions of national social states, from the viewpoint of social work, is the changed social developmental force. This goes hand in hand with a highly charged political change—indeed, each is conditional on the other. The social state is becoming increasingly reduced to the repressive dimensions of the politics of order and control. "The post-social state regulation of social problems is one in which it is not a question of the redistribution of resources and the guaranteeing of rights, but of a 'politics of behaviour'; an ethos politics for the changing and production of attitudes, life plans and lifestyle practices" (Ziegler 2008: 173).

Lessenich (2008) suggests a complex approach to this question. His argument focuses not only on welfare cuts, social privatisation, and regressive state policies in European countries, but also—from a dialectical perspective—raises questions about the shift of societal exchange relationships in which the social complex is embedded. In a historical-sociological discourse analysis, he shows how the social state's programme of practical politics, "by converting numerous institutions of the social state into enablement agencies for active self-responsibility" (84), is already being implemented in many European countries. The relationship between individual, state, and society is undergoing a major shift. "Where once there was public protection of the individual against social risks, [ . . . ] there is now individual risk-provisioning in the interest of society" (95).

Thus, we are not simply talking about political control in the form of reorganisation of the social state, but about a new governmental order of the social—one which is compatible with the demand for flexibility from global capitalism. Social regulation no longer takes place principally through the social state, but through the activation of all citizens, including those who are unemployed or retired. For Lessenich, the activating programmes for 'lifelong learning,' related to the politics of the labour market and education, represent the core of an activation policy in which "institutional strategies and individual ways of acting" merge into a "new form of government of the social (in the broader sense)" (ibid.: 116).

The social state is becoming a socio-technological medium, which keeps citizens on the move in such a way that they do not become a burden on the state and, if possible, generate a surplus that will benefit the common good. The social state is then reduced to the function of regulating this surplus in a community-oriented manner. It is no longer the old model of social state regulation of collective demand and collective feasibility, but one of self-interest with a community-oriented surplus. This correlates to a view of humanity in which *both* "market-oriented *and* socially acceptable subjects" (ibid.: 85) are created *at the same time.*

It is not, however, about returning to the concept of the 'old' nationally bound social state, but about seeking new dialectics and balances in the relationship between the economic and the social—now against the background of local, national, *and* transnational structures. The heart of this reflexivity must be, in our view, that we rid ourselves of the notion that the national social state was and is the only institutional form of the socio-political. Rather, the national social state is *one*—historic—form of the institutionalisation of the *socio-political*, which was formed in the dialectic of the development of industrial society, in the conflict between capital and labour of the late nineteenth and the early to middle twentieth century. In the discussion about the future of social policy as a socio-political framework of social work, we are therefore asking not about the fate of the national social state, but about how social policy today is being set free in new and different ways and what transnational perspectives are being thereby opened up for social work.

## THE CAPABILITY APPROACH AND SOCIAL WORK

An approach that can claim for itself a transnational socio-political perspective of understanding is what is known as the *capability approach.* We propose to use these discussions of the capability approach to indicate the challenges of a socio-political understanding of social work in the transnational context. With the capability approach, a number of different developmental possibilities will be considered and social inequality with respect to individual opportunities will be objectively measured. It is a model that is not limited by national and social state boundaries, but conforms to transnational processes of socialisation. At the centre is the ideal of a *good life,* the attainment of which must be measured by the relation between opportunities of realisation and barriers to such opportunities.

In general, the capability approach developed by Sen (1999) in the last third of the twentieth century today has become the credo of development politics in the transnational fight against poverty. The approach can be briefly defined as attempting to establish a connection between the resources within human beings and what they can (or could) make of them. It is embedded in a programme for the 'good life,' in which, in a spirit of democratic understanding, everyone aspires to primary goods in a globally shared understanding of humanity (approximately analogous to that of the Convention on Human Rights). Sen stresses that the attainment of these primary goods is not only envisaged in the longer-term perspective; rather, it is necessary to tap the individual abilities that might help to bring it about, "the relevant personal characteristics that govern the conversion of primary goods into the person's ability to promote her ends" (Sen 1999: 74). Central here are the degrees of freedom available to achieve the desired end: What options do I have to make something of what I have in me? How can I develop and implement the options for a good life for myself? A prime example of this is the lack of availability of an exit option for women in many regions. Can they achieve the freedom to opt, in principle, for an autonomous life outside gender-hierarchical family structures?

A fundamental feature of Sen's argument is that he looks closely not only at individual diversity of lifestyle, but also at the deviations from the prevailing social norm, and sees that societal institutions are oriented towards a socially conformist average of the population and that they therefore consider conditions of life and lifestyle patterns that deviate from this not as resources but as liabilities. Here the argument comes close to the paradigms (established in social work) of destigmatisation, of empowerment, and of reframing (seeing the strengths behind imputed weaknesses): "With adequate social opportunities, individuals can effectively shape their own destiny and help each other. They need not be seen primarily as passive recipients of the benefits of cunning development programs" (Sen 1999: 11). "(They are) active agents of change, rather than ( . . . ) passive recipients of dispensed benefits" (Sen 1999: xiii). Social work, however, has always pointed out that resources are not simply present in the human being, waiting to be retrieved, but they must be enabled to develop and be socially liberated.

## THE SUBJECT AS TRANSNATIONAL FIGURE OF UNDERSTANDING

Ultimately, in the capability approach, subjective opportunities of realisation become a transnational structure of understanding, and an idea of subjective freedom is universalised. From the perspective of social work, the question is asked whether the idea of the subject having control over itself can be correspondingly universalised. The fundamental question of 'what chances do people have of leading the life that they would like to lead?' (cf. Sen 1999) is based on the premise that those concerned have their own subjective goals to realise, and can be motivated and supported from the outside to realise them. In contrast, social work addresses the question of people's differing life situations and the way they cope with everyday life and the everyday care problems that arise from the ambivalences of their situation in life. Seen in this light, social work always points to the different dynamics that people grasp for themselves when they are subject to the daily pressure of social conditions and are in a care situation: the dialectic of wish and denial.

Of course, we can state that all persons desire a good life for themselves—this is accepted as an anthropological axiom; but the subjective perspectives of development and denial frequently do not meet on the same level. There are social dynamics in operation that lead to the rise of ambivalent constellations in subjective schemes; these can be dealt with individually but are regularly ignored by universalised subjective ideas and approaches to enabling. Thus, social services amount to nothing if they are not founded on the experience of coping with everyday life (Lebensbewältigung).

With Georg Simmel we could ask the broader question whether, in the reception of the capability approach, the focus is on the poor themselves—their coping with everyday life and conditions of care—or on those who are supposed to enable them. In his classic essay on the poor, published over a hundred years ago in 1908, Simmel wrote that the individual poor person was not important for the support system for the poor. "The fact that someone is poor does not mean that he belongs to the specific social category of the 'poor'. [ . . . ] It is only from the moment that [the poor] are assisted [ . . . ] that they become part of a group characterized by poverty." Coser (1977: 182–83) wrote in his interpretation of Simmel, "Once the poor accept assistance, they are removed from the preconditions of their previous status, they are declassified, and their private trouble now becomes a public issue. The poor come to be viewed not by what they do [ . . . ] but by virtue of what is done to them." Community "creates the social type of the poor and assigns them a peculiar status that is marked only by negative attributes, by what the status-holders do *not* have."

This perspective seems to be repeated on the transnational socio-political scale. By the criterion of poverty, societies, or their leading strata, confirm their ideas of freedom and their subjective ideas of realisation as a policy of enabling. They reflect their idea of a transnational world order in the concept of the 'capability approach.' Poverty and social inequality are seen together—in people. From the socio-historical point of view, however, these are different threads of discourse. The social inequality discourse was always a conflict discourse, whereas the poverty discourse was a regulation discourse. Yet it is precisely the tension between regulation and social conflict that has defined the socio-political discourse of social work in the twentieth century and constituted its grounding.

Moreover, in order to be able to address the question of the 'societal opening up' of opportunities for realisation, the capability approach would have to be able to offer a historical and societal theory of development and enabling of life chances:

> The unit according to which, following the capabilities approach, social justice and welfare can be measured, is the sum of actors' enablements and opportunities for realisation opened up by society, i.e. the abilities and power potentials to enable them to realise their intentions and goals. Thus public practices of education, training, support etc. can be

described as 'political and economic' practices, if political economy is understood in the classical sense of (collective) production and provision of goods that citizens need in order to achieve a good life. (Oelkers, Otto, and Ziegler 2008: 87)

It is precisely here that it becomes clear that the concept of the capability approach is moved out of the socio-historical and developmental context in which it was created in the 1970s and 1980s and into the different regional welfare-political discourses, as well as being universalised in terms of welfare policy. Sen developed the concept in a socio-historical and socio-political landscape in which a socio-political development like that of European industrial society was inconceivable. As with the Human Rights Charter, what was important—if there was no prospect of collective social processes—was to be able to make social development perspectives, beyond merely the daily struggle to survive, symbolically visible and attainable for individuals. Freedom for people to shape their own lives is the goal.

Opportunities for realisation are discussed in various contexts and grounded in everyday conflicts and problems. From the point of view of social policy, the concept of the capability approach continues to adhere to a programmatic approach, because although for it society is called upon to make the aim of its social policy the development of a better life for the members of society, similar to the policy of improving life chances in 1980s Europe, Sen emphasises democratic participation discourse, albeit in a rather unspecific manner, and overlooks the developmental dynamics of historical and social structures. Thus the socio-economic question of power cannot be debated.

## STIMULI FOR TRANSNATIONAL SOCIAL WORK

If, then, with this criticism in mind, we ask which transnational challenges for social work become clear in the discussion of the capability approach, two perspectives stand out: the normative perspective and the agency perspective. The capability approach is a *normative* concept. It sets goals for a 'good life,' which comprise socio-anthropological basic figures and contents of internationally agreed human rights. Nussbaum (1999) has developed a corresponding catalogue of qualifications for a 'good life.' Sen is against hard and fast specifications; he prefers, in principle, to leave the choice of goals to individuals or for goals to be agreed in democratic discourse. At issue is the freedom of the actor and his options. However, "the absence of a definition of what makes up a good human life crucially [weakens] the normative force of the capability approach" (Steckmann 2008: 106). Nevertheless, we can see how difficult, even problematic, it is to combine universally and collectively grounded aims with individual ideas of a 'good life.'

From the point of view of social policy, what we have here is a free-floating programmatic approach, as its aims and the opportunities of achieving them are not grounded in the socio-historical and socio-structural conditions and social conflicts under which they can develop and in which they can be experienced. Heimann (1929) addressed this question by looking at the dialectic of the relationship of economic and social development and social ideas. This is why we prefer the concept of the 'better life' rather than that of the 'good life,' because it can ground the normative horizon to the socio-empirical conditions of the current life situation.

It should, of course, be pointed out that the normative horizon only becomes clear for the affected persons when they get the chance to *experience* the fact that they are affected, whether it be in the perception of contrasts with a better life or in the experience of alternative possibilities. In the practice of social work, it is therefore argued that it is not cognitive enlightenment but the offer of 'functional equivalents' encouraging self-value, recognition, and self-efficacy that promises a change in normative attitudes (cf. Böhnisch 1997). Only when social alternatives experienced in this way are present can normative guidelines take effect. This is true of human rights every bit as much as for the principles of a 'good life.'

The *actor's perspective*, which the capability approach especially claims for itself, is also embedded in the aspiration towards the capacity for action. Here, critical reception looks for a link with socio-political debate on agency. Agency is understood as the capacity of individuals or groups to become effective in their environment, e.g., to participate actively in social networks and support groups in order to be able to gain active social control of themselves and their social environment (cf. Homfeldt, Schröer, and Schweppe 2008). Agency as *capability for action*—as the concept is understood in the capability discourse—forms part of a model of expanded capacity for action in coping with everyday life. This becomes clear if we consider the attempts to find a theoretical link with the capability approach based on socialisation. "From the perspective of socialisation theory, the key question is how individuals experience and interpret their conditions of life and what possibilities for action and creativity they offer" (Grundmann 2008: 132). Capability for action—it is said in this context—depends on the experiences of efficacy that a person has had. Whether the experience is of powerlessness to act or of the power to act, "Capability for action is thus directly connected to the evaluations of action and the material limitations or possibilities that prevail in the conditions of life and the social life situation" (ibid.: 137).

These perspectives link directly with the classic body of knowledge underpinning social work. They have no need of the discourse surrounding the capability approach. In many models of social work it is argued that learning experiences develop in which, against the horizon of a 'better life,' the aspiration towards capacity for action is ultimately grounded in the daily accumulation of experiences of coping.

## NEEDINESS AND ITS TRANSNATIONAL
## SOCIO-POLITICAL REFLEXIVITY

We began by speaking about the three Cs: care, commons, and citizenship, which are currently being released in the field of tension between transnationality, the national state, and locality. Care, commons, and citizenship appear as socio-political vanishing points, no longer as reference factors of social work linked in with the social state. In all three dimensions it is evident that suffering in and through society is being socially redimensioned. Here, it is about the socio-historical contexts and, finally, also about how people can experience constellations of need in their life situations and socially transform them. The strategy of setting and hierarchising needs—the traditional business of social psychology—comes into effect again transnationally in the capability approach. The only difference is that here the capability aspect and therefore the development aspect are stressed. However, the approach remains undialectical, as, from the empirical point of view, it is the simultaneity of needs development and denial that can make humans incapable of action.

We attempt to express this constellation of inwardly self-contradictory simultaneity with the concept of neediness (Bedürftigkeit). Many of the problems of coping with everyday life that people in an affluent society have—a society which permanently generates needs, but where the ability to satisfy these needs is distributed in a socially unequal manner—can be summed up in the paradigm of neediness. Transnational processes of socialisation, however, generate a new dialectic of neediness.

There is therefore little point in asking about the 'true needs' that people ought to have or could have, with which the aims of support and intervention ought to be brought into line. Thus those engaging in capability discourse very readily speak of 'deformation of personal self-determination,' by which is meant that "a person [can] find him- or herself in ignorance of what his or her real needs consist of" (Steckmann 2008: 100). In this context they introduce the concept of "adaptive preferences," which seems to imply that people adapt to inhumane conditions—sometimes unconsciously, but also, not infrequently, consciously—thereby accepting that this will involve a "deformation of personal self-determination" (ibid.).

Social work has always been accustomed to such adaptive constellations. But it will not get through to its addressees if it attempts to do so by means of a declaration of right needs and a stigmatisation of wrong ones. We therefore need a conceptual framework for a future, transnationally reflexive form of social work, which is not offered to people from an external source but is derived from the socio-historical and socio-structural developmental conditions of the relevant social conditions of life—and which does not leave it to individuals to decide how to recognise and develop their abilities. Individual patterns of coping have their biographical particularity, but in their fundamental structures they are grounded in the socio-structural conditions of the life situation and the scope such conditions provide. These, in turn, arise from the particular socio-historical development—in the dialectic of expansion or contraction.

## BIBLIOGRAPHY

Baltodano, A. P. (1999) 'Social Policy and Social Order in Transnational Societies.' In *Transnational Social Policies*, edited by D. Morales-Gómez, 19–41. London: Earthscan Publications.

Beck, U. (2007) *Weltrisikogesellschaft*. Frankfurt a.M.: Suhrkamp.

Böhnisch, L. (1997) *Sozialpädagogik der Lebensalter*. Weinheim und München: Juventa.

Bolz, N. (2005) *Blindflug mit Zuschauer*. München: Fink.

Bourdieu, P. (1997) *Das Elend der Welt*. Konstanz: UVK, Univ.-Verl. Konstanz.

Coser, L. A. (1977) *Masters of Sociological Thought: Ideas in Historical and Social Context*. 2nd ed. New York: Harcourt Brace Jovanovich.

Fraser, N. (2009) *Scales of Justice. Reimagining Political Space in a Globalizing World*. Cambridge: Polity Press.

Grundmann, M. (2008) 'Humanökologie, Sozialstruktur und Sozialisation.' In *Handbuch Sozialisationsforschung*, edited by K. Hurrelmann, M. Grundmann, and S. Walper, 173–82. Weinheim, Basel: Beltz.

Heimann, E. (1929) *Soziale Theorie des Kapitalismus. Theorie der Sozialpolitik*. Tübingen: Mohr.

Homfeldt, H. G., W. Schröer, and C. Schweppe, eds. (2008) *Soziale Arbeit und Transnationalität. Herausforderungen eines spannungsreichen Bezugs*. Weinheim und München: Juventa.

Jones Finer, C. (1999) *Transnational Social Policy*. Oxford: Blackwell Publishers.

Lessenich, S. (2008) *Die Neuerfindung des Sozialen: der Sozialstaat im flexiblen Kapitalismus*. Bielefeld: Transcript-Berlag.

Morales-Gómez, D. (1999) 'From National to Transnational Social Policies.' In *Transnational Social Policies*, edited by D. Morales-Gómez, 1–17. London: Earthscan Publications.

Nussbaum, M. (1999) *Gerechtigkeit oder das gute Leben. Dt. Erstausgabe*. Frankfurt a.M.: Suhrkamp.

Oelkers, N., H.-U. Otto, and H. Ziegler (2008) 'Handlungsbefähigung und Wohlergehen: Der Capability Ansatz als alternatives Fundament der Bildungs- und Wohlfahrtsforschung.' In *Verwirklichungschancen und Befähigungsgerechtigkeit in der Erziehungswissenschaft. Zum sozial-, jugend- und bildungstheoretischen Potential des Capability Approach*, edited by H.-U. Otto and H. Ziegler, 85–89. Wiesbaden: Verlag für Sozialwissenschaften.

Sen, A. (1999) *Development as Freedom*. New York: Knopf.

Simmel, G. (1908) *Soziologie. Untersuchungen über die Formen der Vergesellschaftung*. Leipzig: Duncker & Humblot.

Staub-Bernasconi, S. (1998) 'Soziale Arbeit als Menschenrechtsprofession.' In *Profession und Wissenschaft Sozialer Arbeit*, edited by A. Wöhrle, 305–32. Pfaffenweiler: Centaurus.

Steckmann, U. (2008) 'Autonomie, Adaptivität und das Paternalismusproblem.' In *Capabilities—Handlungsbefähigung und Verwirklichungschancen in der Erziehungswissenschaft*, edited by H.-U. Otto and H. Ziegler, 90–115. Wiesbaden: Verlag für Sozialwissenschaften.

Ziegler, H. (2008) 'Sozialpädagogik nach dem Neo-Liberalismus.' In *Soziale Arbeit nach dem sozialpädagogichen Jahrhundert*, edited by B. Bütow and K. A. Chassé. Opladen: Barbara Budrich.

# Part II

# Transnational Social Support and Transnational Organisations

# 4 Development Cooperation as a Field of Transnational Learning[1]

## Kay E. Ehlers and Stephan Wolff

## LEARNING IN INSTITUTIONAL SECTORS

The perpetuation of interorganisational learning depends on the shared learning interests of cooperation partners on one hand, and on interorganisational learning barriers on the other. Learning in and from complex institutional arrangements cannot be regarded—or only to a very limited extent—as the consequence of the efforts and successes of the participating actors. The systematic reference to the deep structures and process rules of the organisations involved is therefore essential for the theoretical reconstruction and the empirical research of learning. The conditions and possibilities of organisational and interorganisational learning (or lack of learning) can only be revealed against the background of those institutional specifics (cf. Ingram 2002). In this chapter, we will attempt to trace this issue using the example of development cooperation (DC). Learning in this large sector is (or should be) an indispensable condition closely linked to both the sector's transnationalism as a set of organisational arrangements and effective social support in developing countries: Which types of organisational set-ups perform better than others? Which lessons have to be learned about successful and failing strategies? However, first of all the problem to what extent organisations and individuals are motivated to learn needs to be analysed.

DC is perceived as the bridging, if not the abolition, of blatant differences of an economic, social, cultural, or spatial type. To this extent, it transcends a goods market, where the defined goals of the organisations involved are to some degree effectively and reliably fulfilled in the exchange of goods/services for money. Hardly anything exists that cannot be the object of DC. Processing decisions and actions in DC, moreover, are much more broadly defined than the repertoire of a single functional relationship (health care, education/training, economy, etc.). Further, DC is characterised by the considerable diversity of the organisations participating in it: consulting firms with profit-making intentions, non-governmental organisations, bureaucracies of the developing countries, development banks, construction companies, UN organisations, village self-help groups—all come into contact with one another.

For this reason it is difficult in DC to implement a generally binding purview of meaning beyond the customary harmonistic rhetoric. A theoretical conception of such complex interconnectedness is intended by the neo-institutional concept of *societal sector* (Scott and Meyer 1991: 117 ff.). A sector means here a collection of organisations in a certain social area, which make a contribution to the production of certain goods or services, or influence the central organisations that produce these goods and services. Functional and institutional aspects, rather than geographical ones, are crucial in the definition of the limits of a sector.

Learning cannot be conceived of as an accumulation of knowledge and ability accessible to all the actors in that sector. A sector is in certain ways integrated. Without question there are common points of reference, global objectives, and binding modes of language. However, there also are—unavoidable in such an extensive ensemble—organisational peculiarities of the most varying kinds. Luhmann (2000: 409) writes of the "contradictory unity of interdependence . . . while at the same time organisations have symbiotic relationships with one another." The conditions of a sector and the interorganisational relationships linked with these conditions create a certain structural resistance against impulses towards change and limit stimuli to learning. Therefore, interorganisational relationships are certainly not fields of learning par excellence. The organisation of learning and knowledge is subject here to a selection that, to a large extent, only arbitrarily favours the declared objectives of development. Between the world of the target groups and that of the strategic decision-makers, a barrier arises that impedes learning processes with diverse organisational 'impurities.'

The general background to interorganisational learning in development cooperation outlined in the following discussion draws upon the results of an empirical study on the sectoral manner of functioning of development aid projects (Ehlers 2011). The four medium-sized projects discussed here lasted several years, were financed by West European development banks, and took place in different West African states from the mid-1990s on. Their common objective was the improvement of access to drinking water and to basic sanitary supplies in selected regions and cities. Different actors from various organisations of the DC sector participated in the measures aimed at hygiene education, water marketing, organisation development, and the building of simple sanitary infrastructure.

These organisations included consulting firms from European industrial countries and local consulting firms, donor organisations and development banks, as well as the responsible administrations, departments, and offices of ministerial organisations or of the provincial government. These vastly diverse organisations, each of them grounded in their own contexts, and their collaboration occurring in an organisationally specific transnationalism, form the core elements and processes of project-based development cooperation. This fundamental structure has to be complemented with other, more peripheral organisations and actors. They include other donor organisations from the same sector operating in the same recipient country, non-governmental organisations with or without administrative backing, as well as 'traditional' structures such as tribal chiefs and clan councils. Furthermore, there are influential individuals (such as local politicians) whose organisational anchoring is unclear, but who have been attributed competence and/or importance. Finally the target group's elements are paramount and must not be forgotten according to the claims and programme. They may consist of neighbourhood communities, villages, or the beneficiaries of training programmes.

This organisational complexity is augmented by substantial differences or even antagonisms between individual persons or departments within the organisations. For example, European consulting firms also employ citizens of the recipient countries at the expert echelon, though less at the executive level. Moreover, one often confronts conflicting interests (or reciprocal deficits in observation) in the administrations of the developing countries, e.g., between government bureaucrats and those from offices in the provinces. Finally, one has to take into account evaluations, either from commissioned evaluators or from delegations from the donor organisations.

## THE RIDDLE OF BLOCKED LEARNING IN DEVELOPMENT COOPERATION

The question of whether and how DC can learn from its own experience in order to improve its performance or performance ability remains open today (cf. Wright and Winter 2010). This is surprising, since in the debates of the 1980s on *aid effectiveness*, donor organisations as well as their partner organisations in the recipient countries were advised to pay more attention to organisational learning. The self-proclaimed transformation of the World Bank into a "Knowledge Bank" by its president during his inaugural address in 1996 lent the so-called *knowledge and learning approach* additional prominence, laying the foundation for today's dominant idea of development aid based on knowledge and learning (Ramalingam 2005).

Nevertheless, the assertion by Cassen et al. in 1986 still seems to apply: The question remains unanswered of whether and how international development cooperation can systematically derive from its experience the capacity for the purposeful improvement of its future performance. Typical actors such as representatives from SADEV[2] self-critically admit that in the field, "despite increasingly rigorous feedback systems, development agencies continue to be criticised for their inability to incorporate past experiences. They are routinely accused of learning too little, too slowly—or learning the wrong things, from the wrong sources" (Krohwinkel-Karlsson 2007: 6). Therefore, what should be cleared up is: Who did not learn here and why not?

Those in the relevant field reflect similarly on the issue. Thiel (1998), editor-in-chief of the German journal *Entwicklung und Zusammenarbeit (e+z)*[3] [Development and Cooperation], criticises what he regards as an obvious scandal. On the one hand, he argues, there is hardly an area of politics that is as strongly marked by continuing learning processes as development politics—because of its supposed nature and *raison d'être*. Evaluations (often conducted on the German side by the BMZ[4]) represent one of the most important resources for the scrutiny of the public, which can find out how many of the financed projects were successful. For the participants in the aid process, the results of such evaluations can help to create a better basis for future work. On the other hand, Thiel states, learning is continually hindered in practice, because the development bureaucracy in effect claims that the learning process can only take place inside the bureaucracy, and operates in such a way that the public, instead of being involved in the process, is merely informed of the result.

In other words, Thiel's assessment posits that the aid development bureaucracy learns, but it does not allow the public to participate in this learning. By withholding a series of evaluations, the BMZ consciously—or at least negligently—hinders the learning of other participants. He detects an inbred or accepted lack of transparency, the elimination of which is increasingly called for by the recipient countries. Why does such obfuscation arise? Thiel's criticism, born of long experience, can be summed up in four assumptions:

*Assumption 1:* No one wants to admit to the uncomfortable truth that single projects have only a slight effect on the development of a country.

*Assumption 2:* Talking about projects and their results becomes too abstract and incomprehensible to the various *stakeholders*.

*Assumption 3:* International aid in developing countries has bred a new parasitic clientelism, centred on intermediaries, the so-called development agents, who can only exist because they understand this jargon and take advantage of it, but who have no particular interest in the successful realisation of projects and their evaluations.

*Assumption 4:* The government ministry in charge exerts pressure on its employees to not reveal details of their knowledge, with a view to either avoid demonstrating political weaknesses or in order to reserve for itself the prerogative of interpretation vis-à-vis other institutional colleagues.

These assumptions imply that, with the good will of all those involved, DC could in fact be effectively designed not just as regards its objectives, but also as a learning process. They likewise signal where one should begin in order to truly make DC a learning relationship between organisations:

*Premise 1:*       Even if deficits of effectiveness prevail at the national level, there are still single projects that work well time and again. Such projects could be multiplied and transposed to the national state level.

*Premise 2:*       If incomprehensible jargon prevents the diffusion of knowledge, the authors of project reports and evaluations could be taught to write more clearly—e.g., at special training courses. It is also conceivable to produce different versions of the same document aimed at specific target groups in order to achieve better understanding among the actors involved.

*Premise 3:*       Insufficient implementation could be corrected by good management, by *good governance* and the exclusion or significant reduction in intermediaries.

*Premise 4:*       A more relaxed attitude of the organisation in charge would be conducive to making the *knowledge and learning approach* more open and dynamic via honest public relations work.

Observers of the political situation in development cooperation must be perplexed that complaints about the alleged learning deficiencies of DC have been lodged in identical form literally for decades, in spite of the notorious denunciations and apparently available corrective measures. Such persistent complaints indicate that when one attempts to comprehend the phenomenon, traditionally assumed causes (such as ignorance, lack of education, political calculation, or scarcity of resources) do not bring one further. Instead one has to change perspectives, i.e., *re-specify* the problem. This is what we would like to do, by describing and analysing the criticised learning barriers as representing both the expression and the result of a certain organisational arrangement.

## STRUCTURE-GENERATED LEARNING BARRIERS

Learning in the DC sector, whether the learning of individual organisations or of the sector as a whole, is apparently a complex and subtle process, involving objectives and standpoints that are extremely different, difficult to recognise, and that are not easily amenable to form a consensus. To expect anything else would mean disregarding the existing segmentation of a functional relationship in simultaneously operative institutions, as much as disregarding a more understandable division into cooperating and competing organisations. Since learning processes (have to) take place in this framework, wanting (or expecting, or even claiming) to recognise in them a 'pure' or 'strictly objective' occurrence is not very promising. Instead, one should first of all attempt to reconstruct the organisational and institutional conditions under which learning—in a broad sense—takes place in (via/with) development aid projects.

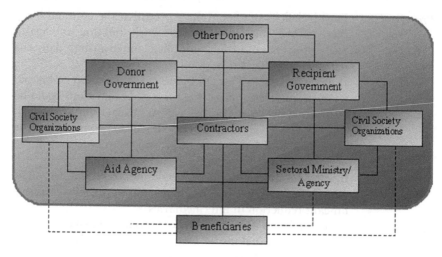

*Figure 4.1* The aid octangle (Ostrom et al. 2002).

Certain types of organisations that operate in the DC sector can be grouped into different classifications. The most prominent modelling of the pertinent interorganisational structure is the 'aid octangle' devised by Elinor Ostrom et al. (2002). As Figure 4.1 demonstrates, one has to expect a specifically accented configuration of institutional players that varies with each DC measure.[5]

Learning processes and knowledge accumulation in the DC sector can be visually rendered and in greater detail using the central sub-processes of the octangle. Three core partners are always essential for the realisation of development aid projects: the donor organisations (or development banks, *aid agencies*), the recipient organisations (for example, state administrations, *sectoral ministries/agencies*), and the consulting firms (*contractors*), whose participation, particularly in difficult enterprises, has hardly been considered in the literature.[6] We would like to now provide a structural illustration, and then use empirical vignettes to illustrate some key mechanisms in the field of learning and knowledge that characterise the exchange between these three types of organisations.[7]

Learning, in the sense of transfer and appropriative transformation of information about innovations, occurs in the interaction among participating actors of the DC sector. From the perspective of observers, this should lead to the build-up of a continuously improved knowledge base and ultimately to changed patterns of action. This optimistic conception of a *cumulative sectoral learning gain* across time can be explained by Figure 4.2.

Figure 4.2 suggests that the knowledge base of the organisations involved (indicated by the size of the circles) increases across time, fed by a constant stream of information (while the intensity of this stream itself demonstrates an increase). The total sectoral system (DC $_{t1}$, DC $_{t2}$), which can be

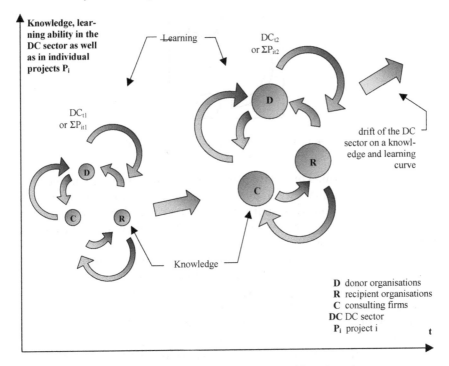

Knowledge, lear-
ning ability in the
DC sector as well
as in individual
projects $P_i$

Learning

$DC_{t2}$
or $\Sigma P_{it2}$

$DC_{t1}$
or $\Sigma P_{it1}$

drift of the DC
sector on a knowl-
edge and learning
curve

Knowledge

D  donor organisations
R  recipient organisations
C  consulting firms
DC DC sector
$P_i$ project i

t

*Figure 4.2* Optimistic conception of interorganisational learning.

conceived of as the sum of individual development aid projects ($\Sigma P_{it1}, \Sigma P_{it2}$), is on a growth path during the course of time (cf. the ordinate indications and the arrows).

The model conception has to be confronted with the particularities of DC practice and tested for empirical validity. We will do this with the help of case vignettes that reproduce typical interorganisational configurations where informing and learning (could) play a role: the reporting back of the consulting firm to the donor organisation on the course of the project ('the report'), the storing of accrued information at the consulting firm ('archive'), the direct exchange of information between all those involved ('the on-site meeting'), and finally the learning of a semantics appropriate to a development aid project by the recipient organisation ('the management of terms').

## THE REPORT[8]

Let us imagine a model conception as shown in the figure of a first key scene of a DC project that is professionally carried out: the learning relationship C >>> D, which is information typically offered to a donor organisation

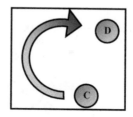

*Figure 4.3*   Consulting firm and donor organization.

by a consulting firm. This relationship is manifested primarily in the periodic (for example, quarterly) *report*[9] during the course of the project. Such reports should not only transmit information. Provided that the characteristic of triggering learning is to be ascribed to them, they should be uncomfortable and irritating, too.[10]

This, however, is not the style in which such reports are customarily written, as the usual term for them used by donor organisations clearly indicates, '*progress* report.'[11] This designation is not an invitation to the author to reveal his or her irritation, criticism of the task, of not knowing how to proceed, or other deviations from the apparently expected normal process of progress. Such a response would constitute for the involved organisations, D and C, an unpleasant, supplementary imposition, ultimately undermining their *raison d'être*. D expects the achievement of the objectives set and does not wish to present itself as the source of tensions and is not designed to process information such as "it doesn't work," but rather to proclaim statements of the type "once more the concept proved itself."

It is therefore necessary, particularly for individual actors who take their responsibility to their own organisation seriously, to demonstrate in these reports that deadlines have been kept, that quantitative objectives have not been fallen short of, or agreements decreed as sensible in the project conception could actually be made. It can make sense to refer to the regular course of a visit by a delegation from the donor organisation, or to an invoice that will soon be due for payment. This specific choice of topics, with its focus on standard procedures, is likely the normal case, but in no way should it degenerate into a triumphal report. Without a doubt there are conditions when this pattern is interrupted, as when the realisation of the project faces serious political resistance.[12] Then learning has to take place or—when avoiding it continues to be advantageous—D has to make increased efforts in order to shield the customary internal patterns from the imposition of an irritation.

The periodical report from C to D ideally signals above all one thing: C does not challenge D with anything other than D's own expectations and claims. D accepts the report; the implied message is that D does not really want to know exactly where the fodder for irritation (from the viewpoint of C) resides. The report is a central act of understanding between C and D;

the report's value resides precisely in its ability to be silent about irritations and to talk about what has been known for long or is at least expected– without bringing in special learning stimulation that seems 'out of context.' Instead, a loose coupling between *talk and action,* in the sense of Nils Brunsson (2003), can be observed. Occasional understanding between these two organisations might even take the character of information hindrance and would then effectively become a learning barrier.

## ARCHIVES

What the organisations learn in exchange with one another represents their growing capacity to operate in the DC sector. That which has been learned must be stored as sector knowledge. This function is fulfilled by organisational mechanisms which can be called *archives*.[13] It does not matter whether such knowledge bases are stored and organised electronically, in paper form, or in another manner. Every organisation which exists in this kind of interorganisational relationship is in one way or another a 'learning organisation.' For the DC sector it is particularly important whether this learning is the result of an organised procurement of new information, or the inevitable, minimum-effort maintenance of established knowledge bases that hardly change. Learning with open objectives can become the precondition for a change in the status quo. But learning can also be adjusted to convenient methods and arrangements, in order to slow down or evade changes.

For organisations of type C two archives are particularly significant. A consulting firm collects all the *reports connected with a project*. This refers not just to the quarterly or to similar reports (*inception report, rapport final*), but also to those documents that had to be produced in connection with the acquisition of the project.[14] These knowledge bases can occasionally simply be copied and used once again for new project documents, particularly in connection with acquisitions. This is a common practice as the conceptual targets in tender documents produced by D (as part of the learning relationship D >>> C not treated separately here) are based on the key terms[15] already mentioned. And these key terms are to be found in the quarterly reports mentioned, which can now be recycled. Archives are not

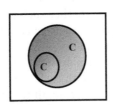

*Figure 4.4* The importance of archives.

searched—and they would be in this sense hardly fruitful—for whether development aid projects have had no impact and have to be considered as failures. An open discussion on the basis of the existing knowledge bases is not carried out. Archives are museums for 'trophies,' with which a consulting firm communicates its functioning in comparable enterprises with the corresponding expert and country-specific conditions.

Just as important is the archive comprised of the *curricula vitae of organisation members*, of those permanently employed at a consulting firm or of those experts hired under temporary contracts. Such personnel constitute an essential component of a bid for a new development aid project during a call for tenders. The personnel archive is therefore much more actively maintained (and is entrusted to specially appointed members of the organisation) than the archive of project reports. One could say that the acquisition value of an expert grows almost exponentially in relation to the duration of his or her missions abroad. 'Experience' is thus rewarded here, too, and consists of learning ways of thinking, keeping deadlines, and using resources efficiently. There is no question that these are valuable characteristics and competencies for experts in a development aid project. No space remains, however, in these curricula vitae for indications of the ability or readiness to explore new paths, that is, for learning in its traditional meaning (cf. Weick 1996). DC is not an area where D, the provider of resources, wants to be unpleasantly surprised. This circumstance is of course known to C and R.

In this organisational context, archives function as strengtheners of the status quo, at least as concerns the area of consulting firms, and as a reassurance for those routines that characterise DC, contributing to an elaborate acknowledgement of "that's the way we have always done it." It is not easy to take or suggest new learning paths away from the burdensome weight of these knowledge bases. At least this would not be possible without the willingness to take risks, and that is hardly to be expected.

## THE ON-SITE MEETING

Since up to now we have only considered learning situations between two of the actors who are involved with learning in an organisation, the question might arise of whether a 'shared learning process' occurs in the form of the joint presence of actors from all the types of organisations at the same time and at the same place, or whether such a shared learning process can be triggered by a kind of 'spontaneous' encounter between the representatives of the different organisations involved. Such encounters are conspicuously rare. Two-sided learning situations clearly dominate, and could result in three-sided learning only through their concatenation across time.

The journey by representatives from all the types of organisations to the *'place of the occurrence'*[16] represents such a three-sided learning event (linked with 'practice'). Not in every case, but often it takes the following illustration:

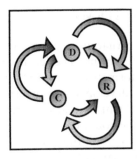

*Figure 4.5* Three-sided learning event.

The D delegation would like to visit one of the 250 villages that profits from a hand pump project to supply drinking water. The village they will visit should be a 'typical' one. A convoy of five all-terrain vehicles sets off and after a one-hour journey arrives in the village. The village might be typical, but of course not the situation. The appearance of the village's inhabitants is by no means authentic, since the project administrators have announced the visit beforehand and an impressive performance has been arranged. Especially popular seems to be attendance of such a delegation to an education course where a 'volunteer,' trained in health and hygienic by the project, holds such a course for the entire population of the village, employing homemade didactic materials. A course with such good attendance has never taken place in the village before; and it will never happen again. The donor delegation, however, is satisfied and R and C are pleased that no 'disasters' have occurred. The convoy can then travel to the nearby provincial capital for lunch.

Nevertheless, even such a contrived event could offer enough material for learning-relevant irritation. The delegation could, for example, discuss with C and R the basis for the volunteer's actions[17] during and after the project. The representative from R could explain the specific political reasons for accepting this specific village in the hand pump programme, but not the much needier ones in the surrounding area.[18] The project head could raise the issue that the modest share of the investment costs, which should have been provided by the village inhabitants, could not be collected, in spite of all the efforts made, and that according to the project's rules, the project was actually not allowed to equip the village with a pump.

Three-sided encounters do not have to take place on-site, but can occur just as well in the conference room of a ministry. They are most often characterised by a broad disregarding of issues that could potentially build up a certain argumentative pressure to change the ways of decisions-making and acting. Although, as mentioned, three-sided encounters are rare, they are nevertheless—particularly and also precisely because of their scarcity—paradigmatic for learning obstruction, and for learning prevention processes in the field of DC. The fear and flight from irritation dominate the scene here in a particularly striking manner.

## THE MANAGEMENT OF TERMS

Another typical learning situation concerns the processing of information in the recipient organisations. The learning recipient organisation is affected by the flow of information[19] from D and C. Projects are not isolated schemes. They have developed out of other schemes, and although they are meant to solve problems or address target groups, they should also have beneficial effects for the donor organisation. Against this background, R takes over *nolens volens* legitimating patterns of argumentation from its 'partners': from D as refers mainly to the strategic targets, from C[20] to the practical management of the process. The representative of R who masters the necessary key terms and the line of thought connected with them, and knows how to enrich them with stories about incidents s/he has experienced, demonstrates that s/he is an expert. Key terms include for example 'participation,' 'decentralisation,' or 'good governance.' R can signal to D and C that understanding will be successfully achieved.

Such a flow of information, whose novelty value quickly diminishes, could in principle flow in the opposite direction, from R to D and C. In view of the distribution of resources and of the idea that it is R, or the field of action represented by R (not D or C), which should develop, this, however, remains a purely theoretical possibility. Judging this constellation might seem difficult, but in the sense of 'self-determined learning' it is not the case. And it increases the probability that the more powerful such a superstructure becomes, the more the objectives and methods focus on sustaining this very superstructure.

A mode of speaking utilising project-sensitive key terms and the corresponding 'thought' can be observed not just at the higher echelons of a recipient organisation responsible at the national level. The same phenomenon occurs just as much in non-governmental organisations, which can be conspicuously close to governments, and among those members of the target groups who have learned to fulfil more or less profitable functions (such as 'agents') in various projects.

A climate of prefabricated discourse facilitates—particularly from the viewpoint of C—the efficient realisation of a development aid project, but

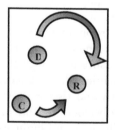

*Figure 4.6*   Behavior of the recipient organization.

hampers the profound understanding of specific conditions and specific project effects. Above all, in such a mental framework failure (and thus the form of learning based on it) is almost impossible; the focus lies on the non-discussable key terms. In the best of cases only tactical learning can occur, a kind of mimicry whose range is limited to the respective occurrence of that project. While D certainly does not want to be irritated by any inappropriate facts in the report written by C (learning relationship C >>> D), in the learning relationships to D and C sketched out here R functions as the ideally irritated one, who feels obliged to state: "Well, that's the way we'll do it now!"

## THE DC PROJECT AS PARADOXICAL TRANSNATIONAL ENSEMBLE

On the whole the phenomenon of 'development aid project' proves to be a highly differentiated hybrid construction. Development aid projects are themselves not organisations, but rather project relationships that extend broadly outwards, for which the term of *transnational ensemble* seems appropriate. As transnational ensembles, development aid projects are embedded in multiple and variable administrative or organisational-political constraints. These involve measures by organisations which hardly know, and are not able to assess, each other. Before they can reach objectives and target groups, they have to come into contact with each other. The *cooperation* between these organisations is successful precisely when their respective forms of existence and their particular logic are *not* fundamentally impaired through the contact, that is, when learning does *not* take place.

The framework for action of the phenomena designated as 'projects' is not produced by the projects themselves. The framework, moreover, cannot be derived from the events themselves; it exists instead as a multiple drawing of borders in the organisations involved. Development aid projects are not self-contained entities that speak for themselves, but rather the intersection of concerns that bring forth an organisational *project occurrence in the narrower sense*, whose basis is precisely not located in an independent project organisation. In contrast, a *project distinct*, 'on-site'-focused, problem-solving concern on the part of the participating organisations and their individual actors is hardly evident. The occurrences constantly lack an overarching inner logic, with the weak inner drive corresponding to the numerous organisational boundaries and graduations.[21]

At the same time, development aid projects are *transnationality in a paradoxical form*. When one leaves the macro level and disregards the embedding of development cooperation work in a political 'one world' rhetoric, then it becomes clear that beneath the transnational surface it is organisations—and therefore *intra-organisational* viewpoints—that dominate. The transnational aspect appears from the perspective of organisations as quite an empty space, only corresponding to the inner logic of participating organisations to a limited degree. One encounters instead an ensemble of organisations, mutually creating the context for each other, which have to cooperate, but can only do this with tactical reservations. Reciprocal adjustment, not orientation, dominates here as the common relationship.

Under such conditions, the repeated call for 'more transparency' can find adherents in the participating organisations[22] only to the point where this recommendation can be sensibly expressed according to the organisation's interests, or to a point from which transparency has to be literally hindered. When it already makes no sense for the organisations involved to grant reciprocal insights into each other, this applies all the more to the 'empty' transnational area mentioned earlier, whose illumination can only be dis-advantageous for all the organisations. The limiting point is marked by the barrier of the *functional lack of transparency*: A complex ensemble such as a development aid project—as presumably DC itself—can only work when one lets the organisations involved have their organisational 'private spheres,' which in no case are capable of communalisation.[23]

In the DC landscape, therefore, a highly professional protection of the status quo flourishes, which hinders stringent learning processes and does not want to recognise the corresponding irritations. In its place, the smooth execution of projects and programmes becomes the uppermost precept of decisions and action. It is thus not surprising that the flows and concatena-tions processed in this ensemble for the most part evade simple (textbook) ideas about 'learning organisations' and 'knowledge and learning based development aid.'[24]

On the whole, a rather pessimistic view of learning presents itself in the interorganisational functioning of DC, in contrast to the first optimis-tic model. The comparison of the two illustrations (Fig. 4.2 and Fig. 4.3) makes clear a cardinal difference: While in the optimistic variant progress in learning and knowledge is assumed for the sector in general (transferred to the ordinates), the more pessimistic and in our opinion more realistic variant displays a *lateral movement* (indicated by the arrows). There is no 'general' growth in abilities and knowledge.

This is noteworthy insofar as the knowledge bases (e.g., the archives) of the individual organisations (with the exception presumed here of only slight growth in R) clearly increase from project to project. However, these knowledge bases—aside from their possible irritating contents of project occurrences—are tailored to the respective functional necessities of the participating organisations (thus, in contrast to Figure 4.2, indicated with a striped surface).

Knowledge bases in individual organisations might increase, but the sys-tem as a whole does not experience a growth in knowledge. Transcending the borders of the organisation and taking in unfamiliar, complex process rules without endangering one's own organisation or other forms of more

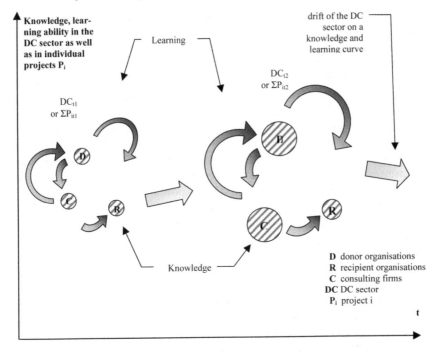

Knowledge, lear-
ning ability in the
DC sector as well
as in individual
projects P$_i$

Learning

drift of the DC
sector on a
knowledge and
learning curve

DC$_{t2}$
or ΣP$_{it2}$

DC$_{t1}$
or ΣP$_{it1}$

D

R

B

C

R

Knowledge

D  donor organisations
R  recipient organisations
C  consulting firms
DC DC sector
P$_i$ project i

t

*Figure 4.7* A more pessimistic view of interorganisational learning in DC.

closely linked knowledge and learning processes have to be regarded as improbable. When both illustrations are compared, it becomes noticeable that the DC system under observation in the more pessimistic variant is substantially more simply structured. What is missing is the feedback of information to D and C from learning situations experienced by R. The system's discursive zone limits itself to D and C.

## WHAT HELPS THE SECTOR LEARN BETTER?

Interorganisational learning is—presumably not just in DC—an exceedingly contingent endeavour, which can easily become entangled in contradictions or remain trapped in dead-ends which at first seemed attractive. One can repeatedly observe that organisations do not use knowledge, which is actually available, nor do they adopt knowledge which is actually learnable, although they could act and make decisions in a more informed and efficient manner. This suggests by inference that *for the organisations* such knowledge can only be considered in a prepared or 'cleaned up' manner. The usual concept of a learning organisation would in fact be that of an organisation which continually irritates itself, which even undertakes that which in the long term it can hardly expect of itself without creating new structures. Such a concept might still work as a programme for small organisations, which operate in a context without strong institutions and with charismatic leadership. In a sector such as development cooperation, however, controlled by large organisations and institutions with a pronounced division of labour, opportunistic learning in the sense of adaptation to institutionalised patterns is much more probable. 'Sectors that learn'—and the more complex the more so—are likely only to remain an idea. Evolutionary change might occur, but not that type of change which eliminates the fundamental problem. Interorganisational learning in transnational relationships or sectors which organise themselves is instead subject to the principle of trial and error, or remains limited to *communities of interest* which spontaneously arise, are strongly dependent on trust and successful reciprocity, and thus not very stable. In any case, it is a slower, much more fragile process than that in a well-oiled bureaucracy with optimised learning strategies. Against this background we would like to finally examine intelligent innovations and irritations that are capable of increasing the structural conditions for learning in such a transnational ensemble as well.

A sort of lodestar for intended change—and not just in the sector analysed by us—is the call for *higher expenditure*, in other words for larger budget shares for DC. Few people in the sector are likely to close to their minds to this demand. It seems, however, not very probable that an increased flow of funds will enable the organisations involved to change their manner of learning. On the contrary, it is more likely that, *ceteris paribus*, the 'margin for error' will become larger, thanks to reduced intra-sectoral shortages and competitive situations.

Similarly, the *improvement of evaluations*[25] or the increased professionalism of the evaluating personnel would initially have one effect: the boom in the sector function of 'evaluation.' It is unlikely that such evaluations would penetrate the organisational structures of the sectors in the sense that these structures—at least partially—are recognised and regarded as superfluous, and instead the needs of the target groups are more clearly considered as the central premise. It would be even more improbable to expect from the efforts put into evaluations anything other than conclusions, and not wide-reaching consequences. Evaluation and learning remain—whether with 'quality improvement' or not—a self-referential act among the organisations operating in the DC sector, since these spare each other mutual impositions as far as possible.[26] The currently highly favoured strategies of context control, in the sense of *good governance*, likewise do not appear very promising in light of the actual existing organisational structures. We suspect that interorganisational learning will free itself even more from replicable project strategies and more detailed process knowledge. Instead, learning itself can focus more on the maintenance of the context as well as on the demonstration of the 'context ability' of the participating organisations.

As regards an answer to the question posed in connection with Thiel's (1998) observations mentioned earlier, whether the premises identified by him could point the way to a development aid practice that learns better, as of now a few cautious assumptions can be put forward. Our diagnosis in this regard is quite sceptical. A sector divided into many players cannot raise well-functioning projects in the sense of a general applicability to a binding 'curriculum,' nor can one expect an eye-opening function from 'clear writing'—what would the actors then see that they cannot already see? It would be more decisive—however (un)clear—to write about the facts beyond the organisational horizons of expectation.

Similarly, we are quite sceptical as regards the strategy of strengthening the learning ability of the DC sector by organisational *re-arrangement of the development agencies*, as it is difficult to understand how organisational arrangements of this kind could avoid the logic and the attachment to the sector. Moreover, as the 'aid octangle' and the illustration of knowledge accumulation (Figures 4.1 and 4.7) suggest, it is simply not enough to locate independent learning, innovative concepts, strategic courage, etc. in the donor organisations. This should be done instead just as much in the other organisations involved.

In our viewpoint a more promising premise seems to lie in the *reorientation of the donor organisations*. Development banks influence the thinking of the entire sector and force learning processes to be oriented towards their perspectives and process rules in the spirit of administrative uniformity. This not only makes DC prone to errors, but also administratively complicated. Development banks should perhaps limit themselves more to that which they undoubtedly do best—namely provide resources (conveniently according to the stipulation of long-term, fixed country quotas)—and content themselves with a function as payment and auditing office.

In this case, the generation of ideas and concepts would have to take place somewhere else, *in the developing countries themselves*. As long as this remains undone in a country or in a sector, this would be understood as a sign that (till now) no substantial demand for the corresponding aid exists, at least none for which a multiplier effect of the development aid project would have a high probability. The demand for resources which has to be linked with such an arrangement should obviously not be expressed haphazardly. The demand for resources articulated on-site should, quite differently from up to now, be directed at an expert competence also located on-site, broadly as independent from the recipient as from the donor organisations. These could be organisations with the will towards organisational independence and a certain code—perhaps such as the Red Cross. Learning and knowledge could then be possibly organised in a manner closer to problems and target groups. On the whole, diversity and ideas competition would noticeably increase. In addition, the apparent failure of concepts necessary for learning progress would have a stronger chance of being possible and recognised.

## NOTE

1. This chapter presents a substantially reworked and enlarged version of Ehlers and Wolff (2008).
2. SADEV: Swedish Agency for Development Evaluation
3. "e+z" is published together with a parallel edition in English: "development and cooperation (d+c)"
4. Bundesministerium für Wirtschaftliche Zusammenarbeit und Entwicklung [German Federal Ministry for Economic Cooperation and Development]
5. By assuming a core of eight types (the category "Civil Society Organizations" appears once on the donor as well as the recipient side) of aid organisations and involving the actual beneficiaries only as the ninth actor, Ostrom et al. (2002) already imply that the flows of information proceeding from and to the actual beneficiaries (represented as dotted lines) are *not indispensable* for the functioning of the total system (which may have to do at least as much with the way 'functioning' is defined as with whether the system 'functions' or not).
6. This division of functions can assume different forms: Non-governmental organisations (NGOs) can take over the functions of administrations and consulting firms, often simultaneously; donor organisations have their own in-house consulting departments; and organisations like the Catholic Church may sometimes assume all three functions in one project.
7. We are concerned here with one selection including the three types of organisations described; we do not claim to reproduce the totality of typical learning situations in DC.
8. In the four development aid projects described in this chapter, reports from the project head level (consulting firm) to the (superordinate) level of the donor organisation constitute a fundamental part of the processing of the project. The reports are expected to accurately and sufficiently reproduce the project occurrences within the period under review. There are regular progress reports as well as a variety of special reports (start reports, interim reports, and final reports). The rule is no report, no project, since the donor organisations can proceed with the necessary actions (for example, payments, authorisations, or approvals) only on the basis of such reports.
9. This report is usually passed on to the recipient organisation (R) or agreed upon with it.
10. The term 'irritation' is used here as an *analytical tool*. Irritation is not used in order to value or appraise something. It indicates a for the moment undefined perturbation which is not compatible with a personal or social system's established expectations (Luhmann 1997: 789 ff.). Effective irritations induce a higher attentiveness but may also lead to surprise, annoyance, or even vexation. Depending on the system and its current condition, an irritation may be very welcomed as 'good news' or firmly refused as "out of standard" (Luhmann 1995: 63). Karl Weick uses in this respect the terms 'interruption' and 'recovery' (thereby referring to John Dewey (1922: 178–79)): "Order, interruption, recovery. That is sensemaking in the nutshell" (Weick 2009: 39). Hence, organisations learn less *from* 'irritations/interruptions' than *due to* them (cf. Christianson et al. 2009), provided the 'window of opportunity' is wide enough open to new knowledge and patterns, i.e., to learning (Tyre and Orlikowski 1994). All in all, the capacity to deal with irritations is a necessary condition for learning.
11. The Deutsche Gesellschaft für Technische Zusammenarbeit (GTZ, German Society for Technical Cooperation) employs such terms. 'Progress report' or 'rapport d'avancement' are common. GTZ has recently changed its name to Deutsche Gesellschaft für Internationale Zusammenarbeit (GIZ).

12. A fascinating episode along these lines is described by Rottenburg (2009).
13. The accompanying sub-illustration cannot be directly derived from the main illustration (Figure 4.2). The concentric circles depict the growth in archived knowledge in the learning relationship C >>> C from the time points t1 to t2.
14. Generally, the 'technical' (expert) bid and the financial bid.
15. C-personnel pay close attention when D-personnel employ key terms in new or repeated ways or noticeably often.
16. As a potential arena for all six conceivable learning relationships, namely D >>> R, D >>> C, R >>> C, R >>> D, C >>> D, and C >>> R.
17. Volunteers who represent a certain promise of sustainability customarily also profit in material terms from projects (in the form of mopeds, T-shirts, or payments) when they make substantial contributions to the project's progress.
18. Doing this would be risky for the R representative; moreover, the questionable practice would continue.
19. Learning relationship D >>> R and C >>>R
20. The organisations encounter each other in a project occurrence via the functionaries typical for projects. On the side of the consulting firm this is the project head, at the donor organisation this might be the country expert, and in the recipient organisation there is the figure of the counterpart.
21. Naturally this does not imply that development aid projects have to always be insipid, or that projects do not lead to results—only that these results often appear to a certain extent 'unofficially' (that is, not mentioned, or only incompletely mentioned in the reports).
22. James March (1994: 64) has no illusions about this as regards other organisations: "The belief that more information characterizes better decisions and defensible decision processes engenders a conspicuous consumption of information. Information is flaunted but not used, collected but not considered."
23. To the extent that sector communication can lead to decisions—for example, in the form of resolutions—then what March (1994: 195 ff.) has described would be valid: "Participants may share some objectives, but characteristically their coalition is a negotiated coalition of convenience as much as it is one of principle. . . . Disagreements are resolved by vague language and vague expectations. . . . Decision makers interested in building viable coalitions are likely to seek and find allies who will be vigorous in supporting symbolic decisions and lax in implementing them."
24. At least it is likely improbable that the requirements of reflection enumerated by Bierschenk (1997: 12) are often achieved: "Thus, whether the actors involved in it are conscious of it or not, development assistance—be it on a national, macro- or on a local, micro-level—is always and first and foremost development policy, and even development politics . . . If every development initiative is an intervention in a complex social game then it might well be worth to find out some essential facts before embarking on it: What is at stake? What are the rules of the game? Who are the main players? Which side do we want to be on? Who will profit from our presence? What is the likely price, in sociological terms, of interfering in the on-going game? Who are we going to hurt?"
25. On evaluations in DC see Schaumburg-Müller (2005).
26. Luhmann (2000: 330 ff.) fittingly writes of the "poetry of reforms."

# BIBLIOGRAPHY

Bierschenk, T. (1997) 'APAD 1996: On the move. . . . ' In *Le développement négocié: courtiers, savoirs, technologies*, Bulletin N° 12, edited by T. Bierschenk and P. Le Meur, 1–5. Hamburg: LIT Verlag.

Brunsson, N. (2003) *The Organization of Hypocrisy: Talk, Decisions and Action in Organizations*. Copenhagen: Copenhagen Business School Press.

Cassen, R., and Associates (1986) *Does Aid Work? Report to an Intergovernmental Task Force*. Oxford: Clarendon Press.

Christianson, M. K., M. T. Farkas, K. M. Sutcliffe, and K. E. Weick (2009) 'Learning Through Rare Events: Significant Interruptions at the Baltimore & Ohio Railroad Museum.' *Organization Science*, 20: 846–60.

Dewey, J. (1922) *Human Nature and Conduct*. Mineola, NY: Dover.

Ehlers, K. E. (2011) *Projekte der Entwicklungszusammenarbeit. Kooperation und Abgrenzung in einem organisationalen Ensemble*. Hamburg: Kovac.

Ehlers, K. E., and S. Wolff (2008) 'Grenzen interorganisatorischen Lernens. Beobachtungen aus der Entwicklungszusammenarbeit.' *Zeitschrift für Pädagogik*, 54 (2008): 691–706.

Ingram, P. (2002) 'Interorganizational Learning.' In *The Blackwell Companion to Organizations*, edited by J. A. C. Baum, 642–63. Oxford: Blackwell Business.

Krohwinkel-Karlsson, A. (2007) *Knowledge and Learning in Aid Organizations. A Literature Review with Suggestions for Further Studies*. Karlstad: SADEV.

Luhmann, N. (1995) 'Die Behandlung von Irritationen: Abweichung oder Neuheit?' In *Gesellschaftsstruktur und Semantik. Studien zur Wissenssoziologie der modernen Gesellschaft*. Vol. 4, 55–100. Frankfurt: Suhrkamp.

Luhmann, N. (1997) *Die Gesellschaft der Gesellschaft*. Frankfurt a. M: Suhrkamp.

Luhmann, N. (2000) *Organisation und Entscheidung*. Opladen, Wiesbaden: Westdeutscher Verlag.

March, J. G. (1994) *A Primer on Decision Making*. New York: Free Press.

Ostrom, E., C. Gibson, S. Shivakumar, and K. Andersson (2002) *Aid, Incentives and Sustainability: An Institutional Analysis of Development Cooperation*. Sida Studies in Evaluation 02/01. Stockholm: Swedish International Development Cooperation Agency (Sida).

Ramalingam, B. (2005) 'Implementing Knowledge Strategies: Lessons from International Development Agencies.' ODI Working Paper 244. London: Overseas Development Institute (ODI).

Rottenburg, R. (2009) *Far-Fetched Facts: A Parable of Development Aid*. Cambridge, MA: MIT Press.

Schaumburg-Müller, H. (2005) 'Use of Aid Evaluation from an Organizational Perspective.' *Evaluation*, 11: 207–22.

Scott, W. R., and J. W. Meyer (1991) 'The Organization of Societal Sectors: Propositions and Early Evidence.' In *The New Institutionalism in Organizational Analysis*, edited by W. W. Powell and P. J. DiMaggio, 108–40. Chicago/London: The University of Chicago Press.

Thiel, R. E. (1998) 'Der geheime Lernprozess.' *E+Z—Entwicklung und Zusammenarbeit*, 12: 307.

Tyre, M. J., and W. J. Orlikowski (1994) 'Windows of Opportunity: Temporal Patterns of Technological Adaptation in Organizations.' *Organization Science*, 5: 98–118.

Weick, K. E. (1996) 'The Nontraditional Quality of Organizational Learning.' In *Organizational Learning*, edited by M. D. Cohen and L. S. Sproull, 163–74. Thousand Oaks: Sage.

Weick, K. E. (2009) *Making Sense of the Organization*. Vol. 2, *The Impermanent Organization*. Chicester: John Wiley and Sons.

Wright, J., and M. Winter (2010) 'The Politics of Effective Aid.' *Annual Review of Political Science*, 13: 61–80.

# 5  New Religious Movements as Transnational Providers of Social Support
## The Case of Sukyo Mahikari

*Wendy Smith*

## INTRODUCTION

Analysis of the functioning of new religious movements (NRMs) as transnational organisations is a relatively new academic field of enquiry (Smith 2008a). Indeed, many NRMs operate in the same way as transnational corporations (TNCs),[1] with the same scale of personnel (members), property holding (centres, headquarters, pilgrimage shrines), staffing issues (posting qualified administrators internationally), budget (donations and sales of spiritual literature and artefacts), and the same transnational, cross-cultural management issues, minus the profit motive. But while the focus of organisational life in TNCs is the maximisation of monetary profit, the focus of NRMs is a spiritual one and their aim is to provide tools, here designated 'spiritual technologies,' for the spiritual development of individuals and the good of the wider society through an ethos of service. It is therefore meaningful to re-examine the research on NRMs for insights into the way they function as providers of social support to their members and others. This chapter will examine the institutions and practices of a transnational NRM, Sukyo Mahikari (henceforth Mahikari), based in Japan, which provides care and support to its members.

After outlining the concept of NRMs and the sense in which they may be considered to be transnational organisations, I will give a brief overview of the movement. Then I will discuss the notion of 'care' and social support in a spiritual context and describe the mechanisms of care in the organisation.

## NRMS—THE PHENOMENON

New religious movements are defined as innovative religious and spiritual movements "characterised by their unconventional symbols of the sacred, their novel understanding of the relationship between the religious and/or the spiritual, and the psychological, their new interpretations of the transcendent, and the new principles of belonging to and/or membership of a religion or spiritual movement which they exposed" (Clarke 2006: 413). The term itself came into use in the 1960s as a way of avoiding the negative connotations of authoritarianism and secrecy associated with the terms 'cult' and 'sect' and, in the West, is generally applied to organisations manifesting in the post–World War II era but may also be applied to movements originating much earlier, for instance, Tenrikyo, founded in pre-modern Japan in 1838, and Brahmo Samaj, founded in 1828 in India (Clarke 2006). Today's mainstream religions such as Buddhism, Christianity, and Islam were new religious movements in their early days, viewed as highly revolutionary by the status quo.

Members of NRMs usually join as individuals who are experiencing hardship in their personal lives, disenchantment with mainstream religious institutions, or economic and social upheaval, such as occurred after the end of World War II or the dissolution of the Soviet Union, where they have mushroomed in its aftermath. Many prominent transnational NRMs have attracted negative media publicity, such as Soka Gakkai, described as using coercive methods to recruit members,[2] and there are some such as Aum Shinrikyo (Tokyo subway sarin gas attack), the People's Temple (Jonestown massacre), Order of the Solar Temple (mass murder/suicide), which fulfill the worst stereotypes attributed to 'cults.'

On the other hand there are those which have a genuine philanthropic agenda in their activities, as well as doctrinal teachings and spiritual practices which aim to strengthen individual well-being within the stress and alienation which many experience in modern urban industrial social life. Institutional arrangements for supporting members in all aspects of personal and social life are often built into their structures and programmes. Indeed, the intense personal help and friendship received in the early stages of contact with the organisation, sometimes termed 'love bombing' (Singer 2003) can be one of the factors in a newcomer's decision to become a member. Once inside the organisation, members may perceive it to be a 'family' which replaces (Ramsay and Smith 2008) or strengthens (Smith 2007a) their existing family relationships.

## NRMS AS TRANSNATIONAL ORGANISATIONS

Transnational NRMs are to varying degrees examined within the literature on transnationalism focusing on diaspora and migration (Levitt 2001; Hirschman 2007), and that of social movement theory, all of which have a potential focus on social support mechanisms at the macro level of analysis. Beyer (1994: 98) notes that social movement theory was a basis for the analysis of emerging NRMs in the 1960s and 1970s. In comparing NRMs with 'new social movements' it is helpful to consider the definition of transnational social movement organisations as akin to international NGOs "who seek to change the status quo on a variety of levels" (Vertovec 2009: 10) focusing on issues which are "transboundary in character, and [ . . . ] draw upon a 'planetization' of people's understandings" (Vertovec 2009: 10, citing Cohen, 1998). Typically NRMs with a transnational presence concern themselves with environmental and health issues and world peace, and have doctrinal elements such as "All humanity is one" (Mahikari), exemplifying the process which Robertson calls "global humanization" (1992).

Mahikari, the transnational NRM discussed here, has a membership of over one million (Inoue et al. 1991) and centres in every continent. In general, all members of NRMs, from every nationality, participate in an organisational culture which often overrides their culture of socialisation or national culture and may, to different degrees depending on the organisation, determine their diet, dress, speech patterns, daily, weekly, monthly, and annual schedules, setting them apart from the mainstream community but linking them in a unique lifestyle which operates transnationally (Smith 2002, 2007b). Members' identification with the NRM as a transnational entity is reinforced by the annual pilgrimages they make to the headquarters of the movement, often an expensive overseas trip.

In the case of Mahikari, unlike some other transnational Japanese NRMs such as PL Kyodan (Nakamaki 2003), the international membership is not at all dependent on the presence of a Japanese diaspora (Japanese members, say, in an Australian Mahikari centre would number around the same percentage as their percentage in the total Australian population; that is, very few).

## SOCIAL SUPPORT IN A SPIRITUAL CONTEXT

In this chapter, I discuss the notion of social support mainly in the sense of the care individuals receive as members of the organisation, but also in the sense of how the organisation cares for humanity and the environment in general. The other context in which NRMs can potentially provide social support is in a diaspora where members use religious organisations as providers of social capital (Vertovec 2000). This phenomenon is typically found in NRMs which proliferate overseas through the migration of their members, which is not the case for Mahikari.

In this perspective I understand social support as "the mechanisms through which a social environment protects its individual members from threatening and impairing events and experiences, and which, in case the latter come to pass and take their course, can support them in their coping efforts" (Nestmann 2005). A NRM can be a total social world for the individual member, providing social institutional frameworks regulating not only ritual and beliefs of a religious nature but also prescriptions for marriage, gender relationships, and wider social relationships, education, health care, economic activities, and the regulation of community affairs normally provided by political institutions. Often the state is in contestation with some of these aspects, for instance, that of medical treatment in the case of the Jehovah's Witnesses,[3] or the education of children in the case of the Brethren,[4] or polygamous marriage in the case of the Mormons.[5] However, when the form these social institutions take does not conflict with wider societal norms regulated by the state, NRMs work within state regulations to provide educational services, health care, counselling, organic food farms, and so on, in other words, a total social environment designed to support members and even outsiders.

The notion of 'community' is used in the special sense of the NRM as a spiritual community, sometimes even designated as a non-kin 'family.' Academic debates on the notion of social support or care have hitherto developed in relation to a need to understand how it takes place at the level of care institutions provided by the state (Daly and Lewis 2000), where the institutional contexts under examination are the family, the community, the market, and the state.[6] The notion of social support also includes 'help' in terms of other voluntary networks (friends, informal networks of association). This chapter contributes a new category to the analysis, that of 'new religious movements,' which can be equated to communities, in the sense of voluntary associations which may or may not have a geographic community aspect in terms of members' proximity to each other, and which, due to lifestyles imposed by the movement, may replace the institution of the family, or the ethnic community, as in a multicultural or diasporic situation, as the group of primary affiliation and loyalty. Certainly it can be seen from the data in this study[7] that membership in these movements can modify the need for members to access state institutions of social support. In that sense, they are an important new institution emerging in the debates on public and private care within the welfare state and on the prominent role of the family as a caregiver. For the purpose of structuring the ethnographic data, Thomas's typology of seven dimensions of care (1993: 656–57)—social identity of the carer, social identity of the care recipient, interpersonal relationship between carer and recipient, nature of care, social domain, economic relationship, institutional setting—is a useful one. The added factor here is that of the spiritual realm, where a transcendent entity may be seen as the ultimate carer, interceding in the relationship between earthly carer and recipient, in the sense that the NRM member as carer is seen as a bodily agent of the transcendent entity, performing the care as 'service' in accordance with the ethos of the organisation. For instance, in the Brahma Kumaris NRM (Ramsay and Smith 2008), if one says 'Thank you' to one of the centre residents for a nicely cooked group meal or other service to members, the person will reply, "Thank Baba" (the Supreme Soul). The idea of a transcendental carer also influences economic relationships and other institutional processes within the organisation. And the fact that the organisation is transnational in its organisational structure and membership means that these mechanisms of social support transcend national cultures and institutions of the nation-state, and are available and accessible to all members from whatever national or ethnic backgrounds, whether at home or while visiting centres overseas or migrating. These dimensions will be exemplified in the case material presented ahead.

## THE CASE OF SUKYO MAHIKARI: TRANSNATIONAL SOCIAL SUPPORT AND CARE

### Origins of Mahikari

Mahikari, often classified as one of Japan's 'new New religions' (shinshin shukyo) (Shimazono 1992),[8] that is, established in the post–World War II era, was founded by Okada Kotama (1901–74), respectfully referred to in the organisation as Great Saviour (Sukuinushisama).[9] In 1959, Okada received revelations from God commanding him thus: "The time of heaven has come. Rise. Thy name shall be Kotama. Exercise the art of purification. The world shall encounter severe times" (Okada 1967). Okada, formerly a member of the Church of World Messianity (Sekai Kyuseikyo), adapted its central practice, Johrei—channelling God's healing light into the body of another—into Mahikari teachings as its main ritual practice, the transmission of Divine Light (Okiyome). When the founder died, conflict arose over who would succeed him. The movement split into two: one group renamed itself Sukyo Mahikari, with headquarters in Takayama, where the Main World Shrine (Suza) has been constructed as a focal point of pilgrimage. This branch of Mahikari is led by Okada's adopted daughter, Okada Keishu, respectfully referred to as Great Teacher (Oshienushisama). The second group, Sekai Mahikari Bunmei Kyodan (World True Light Civilization Religious Organization), retained the original name of the organisation, (note its conceptualisation at the global level of the 'world'), and set up its headquarters in the Izu peninsula. It was initially led by Okada's trusted male associate, Sekiguchi Sakae. Today Sukyo Mahikari has the larger international presence and is the focus of this chapter.

### Beliefs and Rituals

Mahikari beliefs, similar to Buddhism and Hinduism, incorporate the idea of rebirth and the impact of deeds in former lifetimes upon the individual in this lifetime. Mahikari teachings explain that misfortune is caused by malevolent spirits who attach themselves to the sufferer due to karmic relationships created by themselves or their ancestors. The process of purification with the Divine Light pacifies these spirits and causes them to leave the person alone. The result is then a healing on the physical, emotional, or social plane. The bad deeds of oneself (in this or former lives) or of one's ancestors are what attracts the resentment of the spirits of those who have been harmed or their descendents and thus they attach themselves to a victim and cause his or her suffering. Rather than driving these spirits away, in the conventional understanding of exorcism, the process of purification with Divine Light heals them as well and they leave voluntarily.

In Japanese, Mahikari means 'True Light,' signifying the central focus of this NRM, spiritual and purifying energy. It can be partially conceptualised in terms of the concept of psychic energy, Japanese 'ki' or the Chinese 'chi' (McVeigh 1992), but is distinguished by its divine aspect, as the Divine Light of the Creator, Su God. People become members of Mahikari, or kami-kumite (those who go 'hand-in-hand with God'), after attending the three-day training course (Primary Kenshu), a kind of initiation (Hurbon 1991). On completion they receive a Divine Locket (Omitama), which enables them to act as a channel through which they project the Divine or True Light to other members, their families, members of the public, or even animals, food, and localities.

Thus, the Omitama, a spiritual technology in the form of a sacred object, allows ordinary people to perform miracles (Smith 2008b). It is worn on the upper body of members and is treated with great respect. It must not be allowed to become wet or touch the ground. That is why children do not become members until around the age of ten, when they are deemed able to take proper care of the Omitama locket. Members who have received the initial training and have been given an Omitama then have the ability to transmit the True Light following a detailed ritual procedure of praying to the Creator God, which involves bowing to the sacred scroll containing the Chon, symbol of Su God in Japanese calligraphy, enshrined in the Goshintai Shrine, the central feature of each centre, and then to their partner as an act of politeness. Then, with their backs to the Goshintai, they recite in a loud voice, in archaic Japanese, the prayer of purification—Amatsu Norigoto—and Divine Light is transmitted to the forehead of the other person through the raised palm of the hand. Light may then be transmitted to the back of the head and other parts of the body, a complete session taking about fifty minutes.

Giving and receiving Divine Light daily and attending group ceremonies, which are explained as very important to attend as they magnify the transmission of Light from Su God, are the fundamental activities of Mahikari members. Many new members come to Mahikari through being offered Light by an existing member in response to a problem with their health, relationships, or finances. Conversion and care are intimately connected in the case of NRMs as the conversion is usually an individual choice, and individuals entering the organisation are initially impressed by the help and support they receive from members in a very one-to-one sense. In Mahikari, the miraculous healing of incurable diseases such as cancer and the change for the better in relationships and careers, is extensively documented in observably true case histories in the books by Dr. Andris Tebecis (1982 and 2004) (the head of Mahikari's Australia/Oceania division), and in the monthly journals[10] published by the movement. Tales of miraculous reversals of bad fortune abound in the personal testimonies of members which feature in the monthly and annual ceremonies.

## Mahikari Lifestyle

Membership in Sukyo Mahikari organises the lives of its followers quite distinctly on a daily, monthly, and annual basis. In daily terms, as well as giving Light, they are required to offer small receptacles of food and drink to the patrilineal ancestors at their home's ancestral altar, a small traditionally shaped Japanese cabinet situated at head height on a suitable wall. Caring for the ancestors in this way, a practice commonly found in the former rice growing communities of north Asia, as the ancestors provided the grain on which the current generation's food supply is based, is seen as a way of protecting the present generation from harm, in order that ancestors will look kindly on the current generation and not affect the living family or others through becoming attaching spirits with grudges, revenge agendas, etc. Such practices strengthen the cohesion of the family unit. If the Mahikari couple has had the much larger Goshintai shrine, containing a sacred scroll with the Chon, inaugurated in their home, this requires even more care, since it cannot be left unattended for long periods.

There are no dietary codes or dress codes for members, but interaction patterns tend to follow Japanese standards of politeness and respect, and especially in the dojo, removing shoes, washing hands, bowing when passing in front of the centrally placed Goshintai, necessitate mental and behavioural adjustment away from prevailing cultural norms in most non-Japanese societies (Cornille 1991). Gradually one's social interactions tend to revolve around other Mahikari members and membership becomes a total life path. When visiting the Main World Shrine on pilgrimage or other centres overseas, the organisational culture is such that members feel no social or cultural distance between themselves and members of other nationalities. Members from all over the world can be seen giving Light to each other in the universally prescribed ritual style. Thus Mahikari can be said to provide its members with a truly global cultural system (Hexham and Poewe 1997; Smith 2007b). Members have no difficulty in moving transnationally and continuing their supportive involvement with Mahikari as any centre in the locality would be completely familiar to them in terms of its architecture and interior design, its rituals, and the behaviour of its members.

## Organisational Structure and Roles

From its beginnings in war-torn Japan, Sukyo Mahikari has made the transition to a transnational organisation with a clearly defined hierarchy of authority and a sophisticated communication system. Its organisational structure mirrors that of a modern Japanese company, with a Planning Section, Ceremony Department, International Department, etc. At the national level, Mahikari is represented by centres (dojo), which are graded according to their size and importance, from large, medium, small, and associate centres (dai-, chu-, sho-, and jun-dojo), followed by the smaller and more informal 'purification places' (okiyome-sho) and 'communication places' (renraku-sho). This graded system of centres is common both to Japan and overseas. Overseeing the centres are the Regional Headquarters (shidobu), one for each prefecture in Japan, and one each for Europe/Africa, North America, Latin America, Asia, and Australia/Oceania. A shidobu is headed by the division head (Bucho) (a term used for a senior manager in a Japanese corporation) on behalf of Oshienushisama and his role[11] includes both spiritual and managerial aspects; in fact he serves as a major caretaker in the organisation, regionally, and for its members on a one-to-one basis. The Bucho visits centres in all the countries in his region regularly, conducting the Primary Training and bestowing the symbol of membership and the spiritual technology for mutual caring, the Omitama, on new members. He gives Light to members constantly. He also administers the region, overseeing and recommending staff transfers and promotions in rank, and conducts the regional monthly ceremony as the spiritual representative of Oshienushisama.

Below Oshienushisama herself are a few very senior members of Sukyo Mahikari Headquarters. In general the main ranks are Ministers (Doshi) and Centre Chiefs (Dojocho). Centre Chiefs, the status below Bucho, are spiritually in charge of the centre, are usually from the locality and, unlike Ministers, are rarely transferred away from their city of residence and employment. Hence they get to know the local members very well and also perform supportive roles, combining spiritual and secular counselling elements.

## Mechanisms of Care and Support in Mahikari

Ministers are the movement's professional caregivers, although all members are encouraged to give care and support to each other and to outsiders through the practice of giving Divine Light. They are the disciples of Oshienushisama who have undertaken a three-year training course. There are from thirty to fifty new trainees in every annual intake, selected from hundreds of applicants.

Being of all nationalities, Ministers play an important linking role in promoting the transnationality of the organisation and may be transferred, often at intervals of about three years across national boundaries. For instance, a former Minister at the Melbourne centre was South African, there have been two Japanese Ministers serving in the Canberra Regional Headquarters and Australian Ministers have been posted to the International Division in Takayama and to a centre in India.

Within the centre there are different group leaders, coordinators, and other personnel who coordinate such groups as the Parents' Group, Educators' Group, Older Youth Group, Primary Students' Group, Kindergarten Group, and so on. All of these groups are designed to give support with practical daily life issues reinforced with spiritual support to members. As it is believed that the spirit world influences the circumstances of life in the everyday world, spiritual and practical support for problems are intertwined. This organisational ethos of support is reinforced by the ritual exchange of Divine Light between members whenever these groups, and indeed individuals, meet formally or informally. There are also various leadership roles relating to the Yoko agriculture (a horticultural project based on organic and spiritual principles) and medical care facilities run by the organisation. In these systems, spiritual elements and modern bureaucratic principles are combined.

A key social support institution in the movement is the formal role of 'Group Carer.' Created after the membership drop-out rate became a concern, Group Carers, relatively senior members of a centre who have been permitted to install a Goshintai in their homes, look after a small group of members and their families, around ten, acting as counsellors for any problems they might be having and keeping in touch with them on a regular basis. Group Carers are busy giving Light to their members as often as they can. The Group Carer would be the first person to approach a member whose attendance at the centre had diminished, to check if there were any major problems contributing to the decrease in his or her active participation. If a member wished to leave the movement, however, he or she would be free to do so.

The members of a Group Carer's circle usually attend the monthly 'Goshintai appreciation ceremony' conducted for the Goshintai at his or her home. This involves the giving of Light, formal prayers and rituals associated with the Goshintai, then a tea party, to which all have brought contributions of food. Members make offerings to the Group Carer's Goshintai offering box, which will later be conveyed to the main centre. The group centring around a Group Carer provides a very accessible daily life support mechanism for mothers with young families, youth working in a city away from home, divorced or aged members living alone. The mixture of human friendship, social events, and personal counselling found in a Group Carer's group is reinforced with the background of commonly understood spiritual principles which are a frame of reference for advice or interaction, plus the powerful purifying impact of the ritual exchange of Divine Light. It is important to note that giving Light is not an elitist one-way process (members give and receive in turn) but a spiritual act which all who possess an Omitama can perform equally and hence all can potentially serve as agents for positive change in the recipient's health, emotional state, relationships, career, or business success, etc. And the act of giving Light is beneficial to the giver as well. Even in social psychological terms, the opportunity to play the role of benefactor to someone else could be seen as strengthening to the identity and emotional state of that person. Thus through the simple process of attending a three-day training seminar, obtaining an Omitama, and learning the simple ritual of claps and bows, and memorising the ritual prayer Amatsu Norigoto, proclaimed in Japanese by members of all nationalities while giving Light, all members can and do care for each other on a regular basis—potentially and in reality effecting miracles of healing and transformation upon their co-members, and also upon people outside the organisation if they agree to receive the Light.[12]

As well as the community of members clustering residentially around a centre, and the sub-groups focused around Group Carers, Mahikari celebrates and supports the nuclear family as a social institution. The function of the nuclear family as a source of social support is rapidly declining in modern and post-modern society as marriage rates decline and single parent households increase,[13] but Mahikari celebrates members' social identities as members of patrilineal families, in a way very similar to the emphasis on family roles in Confucian societies such as Japan. A feature of all large centres is the provision of a family room where parents can be with small children while receiving the Divine Light or listening to lectures through the installed sound or video system. Members of a family possessing Omitama are encouraged to give and receive Light, to each other daily and also give Light to children and non-members in the family. The focus on the family is further reinforced by the daily food offerings to the ancestors reminiscent of, but not identical to, Buddhist practices in the traditional Japanese household. Mahikari Youth group activities give a role to the children of members within the organisation, and the Youth, in striking uniforms, have key roles in major ceremonies. In NRMs initial membership is by individual conversion. In this way, the organisation attempts to solve the problem of establishing a pattern of intergenerational membership when no wider community traditions are in place, as in the case of Christianity, Islam, or Buddhism, for example, to ensure that children will follow the faith of their parents.

Significantly, this NRM is providing support services which professionals provide in a secular world, that of counselling and psychological support. Financial support is usually not needed by Mahikari members who are mainly working in mainstream occupations and are able to give substantial donations to the movement. If anyone falls on hard times, there would be various spiritual technologies to reverse the situation, giving Divine Light to the business premises, changing one's innermost attitude (sonen), and so on. Converts relate various stories of the miraculous recovery of their financial circumstances after joining Mahikari. If, however, misfortune befalls someone after joining, this is explained as a 'cleansing' in the same way as those receiving the Divine Light may experience strong episodes of vomiting, diarrhoea, or fever, as a cleansing. Many relate how the smell of medicines consumed over decades permeates these bodily incidents, so that they can easily relate the phenomenon of misfortune to that of cleansing.

## Care Beyond Mahikari Membership

Mahikari rituals and practices are also conducted for the good of the wider community and ultimately all humanity. For instance, a basic element in the daily opening ceremony of each centre is for all present to revolve slowly around 360 degrees, reciting the prayer of purification, the Amatsu Norigoto, while radiating Light with raised hands, and thus purifying the neighbouring buildings and environment. Food prepared at home, merchandise, cars, etc. are also purified with the aim of benefiting those who use them.

The organisation provides medical care for members and the wider community at its Yoko Clinic at its headquarters in Takayama, where modern medical treatment is combined with the transmission of Divine Light if the patient wishes to receive it. The hospital has a Mahikari practice centre on the top floor and staff are Mahikari members.

In terms of service to the environment, Mahikari operates a system of ecological farming, in its Yoko Farm movement, where no pesticides are used, and the movement mirrors the holistic farming established by Findhorn. Indeed when one visits the Yoko farms, there are stories of miraculously large vegetables and bumper crops, and also the phenomenon of how pests and predators migrate from neighbouring farms because of the absence of traditional pest repulsion methods.

## THE DARK SIDE OF NRMS IN RELATIONS TO ISSUES OF CARE

In all large organisations, there is the possibility of some members' behaviour being less than ideal in terms of their intentions or practice of the principles. A few individuals may even join spiritual organisations to obtain personal power, or other self-oriented benefits. Usually the lifestyle and practices of NRMs screen out such members and they leave, but when large numbers in the hundreds of thousands are involved, there is always the possibility that some members will be problematic. Indeed many NRMs show evidence of such phenomena and websites of disenchanted members can be found. The Internet has proved to be a powerful tool for former members to air their grievances.

In the case of Mahikari, some disenchanted former members set up a website which has had damaging results for the organisation. Their claims related to financial matters which may have been in a secular business context. Conversion to a new religious movement involves changes in lifestyle, relationships, and voluntary financial outlays in the form of donations, which may be quite considerable in the initial enthusiasm of joining and experiencing new phenomena. When the individual subsequently does not achieve what he or she expected, it may lead to disenchantment. This cycle is well documented in the literature on membership in NRMs.[14] In relation to Mahikari, speaking from my knowledge of the centre administrators, Doshi, and ordinary members whom I met in my research in Mahikari centres in five countries, the impression I received is of dedicated and goodhearted individuals who are living a lifestyle of daily spiritual awareness and gratitude, with the sincere aim of helping other members, society, and humankind in general. The living circumstances of members and Centre and regional administrators are modest and there is no evidence of the opulent display or desire for personal gain, power, and status associated with leadership roles in some NRMs. In fact, the Doshi, who live in centres with very few personal possessions, demonstrate a high level of personal self-sacrifice.

## Conclusion

Mahikari, like many other Japanese NRMs, arose in the 1950s in the context of the devastation of material and economic life in Japan after her defeat in World War II. Individuals were able to obtain help with their health, relationships, and even economic problems through receiving the Divine Light. Hence, in Mahikari, care is primarily in terms of the practice of giving Divine Light, a daily obligation, towards one's family members, at the centre to other members and visitors, and even on the street, if someone is in trouble.

Using the case of Sukyo Mahikari, this chapter applies the notion of transnational social support to a new area, that of new religious movements, and investigates them as providers of a universal system of social support and care to individuals both inside and outside the organisation, in a spiritual way through spiritual means, and in a secular way through their secular, albeit spiritually enhanced, institutions.

In Mahikari, this transnationality is facilitated by the main element of its spiritual culture and also its main mechanism of caring, the ritual practice of radiating Divine Light. This has been a powerful factor in establishing uniformity in the value systems and behaviour of Mahikari members in diverse cultures. This is strengthened through the doctrinal emphasis on purification, especially the process of purification of members' innermost attitude (sonen). Moreover the occurrence of miracles associated with the Divine Light has been a compelling reason behind members' conversion and the main reason for its global spread. Purity and miracles are concepts which transcend different cultures.

The care and support taking place in NRMs such as Mahikari are transnational in two senses: firstly because the care mechanisms are embedded in the organisational culture, which is transnational and uniform throughout the organisation, they can be accessed by any member anywhere in the globe; and secondly, because the organisation actively posts its senior members around the globe to introduce, support, or enhance the service and hence the care practices in the local national centres. These postings are very strategic, with the aim of benefiting humanity in both the spiritual and secular realms—enhancing the spiritual development of members and providing service to the wider society through secular programmes, campaigns with both practical and spiritual effects, and through trying to make inroads into secular institutions through educating public figures about their ideals.

### NOTES

1. Transnational corporations (TNCs), or multinational corporations (MNCs), or enterprises (MNEs) are firms which own or control production facilities or deliver services in more than one country, with headquarters in a home

country and subsidiaries or operating units in host countries. TNCs are distinguished by the fact that they have a more global emphasis in their corporate culture and operations.

2. Shakubuku is a controversial method of propagating Nichiren Buddhism using dialogue to refute another's heretical views. Sometimes translated as 'break and subdue,' it also has the sense of cutting through delusion. However, the methods used by zealous members of Soka Gakkai were sometimes seen as too strident and coercive.

3. Jehovah's Witnesses are not allowed to accept blood transfusions for themselves or their children, believing that this is the same as eating blood and is forbidden in the Bible. Many Jehovah's Witnesses have died because of this restriction the Watchtower Society has placed upon its members. In the past the Watchtower Society has forbade them to get vaccinations or accept organ transplants; many people died needlessly before the Watchtower Society changed its rules and allowed these procedures. They still hold fast to the prohibition against receiving blood transfusions (http://www.towerwatch. com/Witnesses/Beliefs/their_beliefs.htm. Retrieved 27 March 2011).

4. Wilson, B. (2000) "'The Brethren': A Current Sociological Appraisal." http:// www.theexclusivebrethren.com/documents/academicstudy.pdf. Retrieved 27 March 2011.

5. Hardy, B. C. (1992) *Solemn Covenant: the Mormon Polygamous Passage*. Champaign, IL: University of Illinois Press.

6. In developed economies such as Australia, the state supports the family as an institution of care by providing, for instance, 'carer allowances' for children to look after elderly parents at home, child support allowances, 'in the home' domestic helpers, rent relief for the unemployed, etc. In relation to the workplace, there is legislation requiring employers to grant maternity leave, paternity leave, carer's leave, etc. indicating support funded by the market. From a community perspective, for instance, there are church or other religious or secular charities providing accommodation for the homeless, food, clothing, furniture for low-income groups, etc.

7. The author is a social anthropologist who carried out research on Sukyo Mahikari from 1995 to 2001 in Australia (Melbourne, Adelaide, Sydney, Canberra), Malaysia (Kuala Lumpur), Singapore, the Philippines (Manila), and Japan (Takayama, Kyoto, Tokyo, Nagoya) using participant observation, structured and unstructured interviews, and documentary data collection methods.

8. According to Shimazono (1992, as outlined in Reader 1993: 235) the 'new New Religions,' which emerged after World War II and particularly those which have showed dynamic growth in the 1970s and 1980s, are distinguished by a focus on immediate benefit in the here and now in their practices and beliefs and on the abilities demonstrated by the charismatic leaders of the movements. Thus the new New Religions offer tangible benefits and salvation in this world, as opposed to the other-worldly focus of Buddhism. Importantly, in new New Religions such as Mahikari, belief in the purifying power of God's light is linked to ethical systems in a very this-worldly context. New Religions teach that one's fate is not solely determined by the power of God or other transcendent beings, but that one can achieve salvation and happiness in this life by one's own efforts, such as changing one's attitude and daily behaviour (Shimazono 1993: 293). Shimazono also emphasises the importance of the spiritual status of the individual, as opposed to that of the family or the community as in the established religions or folk religion in Japan. In Mahikari this is represented by the belief in an individual's guardian spirit and in individual spiritual advancement.

9. This section is derived from Smith (2007a).

10. For instance, the *MAAJ—Mahikari Australia and Asia Journal*, published by Sukyo Mahikari Australia Ltd.

11. In Sukyo Mahikari, Bucho are usually male, as are senior managers in Japanese corporations.

12. See many accounts of these miracles in the two books by Tebecis (1982, 2004). I conducted this research over a number of years as an anthropologist using the methodology of participant observation. It was a condition of my research on Mahikari that I receive the Light every time I visited the dojo before beginning interviews. In the course of conducting research in this way, I personally experienced the 'miracle' of painful gallstones, visible on an ultrasound scan and which the doctor said needed surgical removal, disappearing after a session in which I received the Light during a fieldwork visit to the Melbourne *dojo*.

13. http://www.census.gov/compendia/statab/2011/tables/11s1335.pdf. Retrieved 29 March 2011.

14. See, for instance Bromley, D., ed. (1988) *Falling from the Faith: The Causes and Consequences of Religious Apostasy.* Newbury Park, CA: SAGE Publications.

## BIBLIOGRAPHY

Beyer, P. (1994) *Religion and Globalization.* London: Sage.
Clarke, P. B. (2006) *Encyclopedia of New Religious Movements.* Oxford: Routledge.
Cohen, R. (1998) 'Transnational Social Movements.' Oxford ESRC Transnational Communities Programme Working Paper WPTC-98–10. http://www.transcomm.ox.ac.uk/working%20papers/cohen.pdf. Retrieved 2 November 2011.
Cornille, C. (1991) 'The Phoenix Flies West: The Dynamics of the Inculturation of Mahikari in Western Europe.' *Japanese Journal of Religious Studies*, 18(2–3): 265–86.
Daly, M., and J. Lewis (2000) 'The Concept of Social Care and the Analysis of Contemporary Welfare States.' *British Journal of Sociology*, 51(2): 281–98.
Hexham, I., and K. Poewe (1997) *New Religions as Global Cultures—Making the Human Sacred.* Boulder, CO: Westview Press.
Hirschman, C. (2007) 'The Role of Religion in the Origins and Adaptation of Immigrant Groups in the United States.' In *Rethinking Migration—New Theoretical and Empirical Perspectives*, edited by A. Portes and J. DeWind, 391–418. New York: Berghahn Books.
Hurbon, L. (1991) 'Mahikari in the Caribbean.' *Japanese Journal of Religious Studies*, 18(2–3): 243–64.
Inoue, N. et al. (1991) *Shinshukyo jiten (Encyclopedia of the New Religions).* Tokyo: Kobundo.
Levitt, P. (2001) 'Between God, Ethnicity, and Country: An Approach to the Study of Transnational Religion.' Paper given at workshop on "Transnational Migration: Comparative Perspectives," 30 June–1 July 2001. Princeton: Princeton University.
McVeigh, B. (1992) 'The Vitalistic Conception of Salvation as Expressed in Sukyo Mahikari.' *Japanese Journal of Religious Studies*, 19(1): 41–68.
Nakamaki, H. (2003) *Japanese Religions at Home and Abroad—Anthropological Perspectives.* London: Routledge & Curzon.

Nestmann, F. (2005) 'Soziale Netzwerke—Soziale Unterstützung.' In *Handbuch Sozialarbeit/Sozialpädagogik*, edited by H.-U. Otto and H. Thiersch, 1684–93. Neuwied. Munich: Ernst Reinhardt Verlag.

Okada, K. (1967) *Mioshieshu (Collected Sacred Teachings)*. Tokyo: Sekai Mahikari Bunmei Kyodan.

Ramsay, T., and W. Smith (2008) 'The Brahma Kumaris World Spiritual University.' *IIAS Newsletter*, 47: 1, 4, 5. http://iias.asia/newsletter-47. Retrieved 2 November 2011.

Reader, I. (1993) 'Recent Japanese Publications on the New Religions in the Work of Shimazono Susumu.' *Japanese Journal of Religious Studies*, 20(2–3): 229–48.

Robertson, R. (1992) *Globalization: Social Theory and Global Culture*. London: Sage.

Shimazono, S. (1992) *Gendai Kyusai Shukyoron [The Study of Contemporary Salvationist Religions]*. Tokyo: Seikyusha.

Shimazono, S. (1993) 'The Expansion of Japan's New Religions into Foreign Cultures.' In *Religion and Society in Modern Japan*, edited by M. Mullins et al., 273–300. Berkeley: Asian Humanities Press.

Singer, M. (2003) *Cults in Our Midst*. Revised ed. San Francisco: Jossey-Bass.

Smith, W. (2002) 'The Corporate Culture of a Globalized Japanese New Religion.' *Senri Ethnological Studies*, 62: 153–76.

Smith, W. (2007a) 'Sukyo Mahikari in Australia and Southeast Asia: A Globalized Japanese New Religious Movement outside the Japanese Diaspora.' In *Japanese Religions in and beyond Japanese Diaspora*, edited by R. A. Pereira and H. Matsuoka, 45–78. Berkeley, CA: UC Berkeley/Institute of East Asian Studies.

Smith, W. (2007b) 'Asian New Religious Movements as Global Cultural Systems.' *IIAS Newsletter* 45: 16–17. http://iias.asia/newsletter-45. Retrieved 2 November 2011.

Smith, W. (2008a) 'Asian New Religious Movements as Global Organizations.' *IIAS Newsletter* 47: 3. http://iias.asia/newsletter-47. Retrieved 2 November 2011.

Smith, W. (2008b) 'A Global NRM Based on Miracles: Sukyo Mahikari.' *IIAS Newsletter* 47: 12–13. http://iias.asia/newsletter-47. Retrieved 2 November 2011.

Tebecis, A. K. (1982) *Mahikari: Thank God for the Answers at Last*. Tokyo: L. H. Yoko Shuppan.

Tebecis, A. K. (2004) *Is the Future in our Hands? My Experiences with Sukyo Mahikari*. Canberra: Sunrise Press Pty Ltd.

Thomas, C. (1993) 'De-constructing Concepts of Care.' *Sociology*, 27(4): 649–69.

Vertovec, S. (2000) 'Religion and Diaspora.' Paper given at the conference on "New Landscapes of Religion in the West," School of Geography and the Environment, University of Oxford, 27–29 September 2000.

Vertovec, S. (2009) *Transnationalism*. London: Routledge.

# Part III
# Transnational Family Care

# 6 Negotiating Double Binds of In-Between

## A Gendered Perspective of Formal and Informal Social Supports in Transnationality

*Luann Good Gingrich*

A French feminist playwright and theorist, Hélène Cixous, writes this about the place of in-between, of *entredeux*:

> Entredeux is a word . . . to designate a true in-between—between a life which is ending and a life which is beginning. For me, an *entredeux* is: nothing. It *is*, because there is *entredeux*. But it is—I will go through metaphors—a moment in a life where you are not entirely living, where you are almost dead. Where you are not dead. Where you are not yet in the process of reliving. These are the innumerable moments that touch us with bereavements of all sorts. There is bereavement between me, violently, from the loss of a being who is a part of me—as if a piece of my body, of my house, were ruined, collapsed . . . Everything that makes the course of life be interrupted. In this case we find ourself in a situation for which we are absolutely not prepared. Human beings are equipped for daily life, with its rites, with its closure, its commodities, its furniture. When an event arrives which evicts us from ourselves, we do not know how to 'live'. But we must. Thus we are launched into a space-time whose coordinates are all different from those we have always been accustomed to. In addition, these violent situations are always new. Always. At no moment can a previous bereavement serve as a model. It is, frightfully, all new: this is one of the most important experiences of our human histories. At times we are thrown into strangeness. This being abroad at home is what I call an *entredeux*. Wars cause *entredeux* in the histories of countries. But the worst war is where the enemy is on the inside; where the enemy is the person I love the most in the world, is myself (Cixous and Calle-Gruber 1997: 9–10).

In this chapter, I seek understanding of places and spaces *entredeux*—in-between settlement and migration, in-between acculturation and separation, in-between nation and culture, in-between inclusion and exclusion. This analysis is part of a larger investigation that explores meanings and expressions of choice and agency, and the paradoxes of self-imposed or voluntary social exclusion within a social service system that promotes a commonsense version of social inclusion as a universal good. A central question guiding this programme of research and the discussion that follows is this: How do we understand and respond to individuals and groups who appear not to choose what is 'good' for them; who resist inclusion, integration, belonging in any measure; whose priority is to preserve the 'foreign' across time and place? My specific focus for this inquiry is the in-between of transnational livelihoods that are made necessary by widening economic, social, and subjective divides, and which require (im)migrant women to navigate and negotiate conflict between competing systems of social support: between, on the one hand, unfamiliar formal social supports, such as various human services in the well-developed welfare state of many destination countries; and on the other, the essential and everyday informal social supports of family, community, and work.

For Low German Mennonite women, family and community are the essence of daily life, work, home, personal and collective identity, and hope. Yet many families are leaving their colonies, or 'sacred villages,' in Latin America in search of a better life. In Canada, Mennonite (im)migrant[1] women describe being confronted with the outside world in ways that are both freeing and formidable, as traditional cultural and religious practices conflict with the values and norms of a society that seeks to lift women out of bondage (Good Gingrich and Preibisch 2010). I propose that migration necessarily involves negotiating contradiction, confrontation, and conflict—contradictions arising in the loss of familiar means of survival; confrontation between incompatible livelihood practices; and conflict between competing values and norms and strategies for getting ahead in spaces in-between. The following is a re-telling of the stories of *entredeux*, of bereavement and strangeness, of interrupted lives. Specifically, through the case example of migrating Low German Mennonite women and their families, I aim to examine the ways in which the family and ethno-religious community, and women's work as vital to these informal social support systems, are adjusted and defended through voluntary and involuntary encounters with formal social supports in these transnational, transcultural—even trans-temporal—migrations. These stories of in-between also bring to the fore the dual and often contradictory functions of formal social supports, in the form of various social services, that despite a pervasive ideological commitment to individual rights and freedoms, demand a high degree of conformity to specific cultural and even religious norms, values, and daily life practices. My overall objective is to inform social work policy and practice with (im)migrant families.

This work is based on qualitative data from three recent research projects, collected through interviews and focus groups with fifty-six Low German Mennonites who migrated to Canada from Mexico or other regions of Latin America, and with forty Canadian service providers and employers who work with this population.[2] These studies concentrated on issues of work or livelihoods, social policy, and social services in the everyday for this ethno-religious group of (im)migrants. I emphasise the uniquely gendered perspective of Low German Mennonite (im)migrant women who maintain varying degrees of transnationality between their colony in Latin America and rural communities in Canada.

Most of the (im)migrant respondents are members of the Old Colony church, the most traditional of the various and diverse Low German Mennonite church groups. Service providers represented a wide range of human services, including employment programmes, child welfare, social assistance (or workfare), public housing, school boards, public health, mental health, and primary health care.

## WRITING IN-BETWEEN

The social relations I describe cannot be escaped, even temporarily. As a social services researcher and practitioner, and as a (Swiss) Mennonite[3] mother, I am neither inside nor outside, up nor down, in the analysis that follows. Insisting on an ambiguous point of view, a consciousness and conscious in-between, I reinsert the research accounts into their social and historical contexts through a reiterative and hermeneutic approach to the data—a process of moving back and forth, between then and now; between what I know from my own life and what respondents told me; between academic socio-historical literature and lived experience. My vacillating vantage point is a self-conscious locating, as I aim to tell the story of (im)migrant women's experience of the transnational on their terms rather than my own. I also resist the familiar presumption of a "bird's-eye view," "a position outside" (Smith 1999: 54), that tends towards judgment while falsely claiming neutrality or even moral superiority. In this way, I strive towards understanding—or at least "positive incomprehension" (Cixous and Calle-Gruber 1997: 16)—of spaces *entredeux*—of in-between—from and through in-between.

## IN-BETWEEN NATION-PLACE

The roots of the Low German-speaking Mennonites from Latin America are religious, originating in the sixteenth-century Protestant Reformation in Europe. A small group of radical reformers became known as the Anabaptists, departing from the newly formed Protestant Church on several points of religious ideology and practice. The central tenets of the Anabaptist movement included believer's (or adult) baptism, the authority of the New Testament scriptures, the 'priesthood of all believers,' or communal scriptural study and shared church leadership, and definitive separation of church and state. Named after Menno Simons who in 1536 renounced the Catholic priesthood and was re-baptised as an Anabaptist elder, the first Mennonites distinguished themselves from other Anabaptists by their rejection of the use of violence, even in self-defense.

Because their radical beliefs and practices directly challenged the religious and political institutions of the day, many Anabaptists were persecuted and killed. Thus, invisibility and movement were vital to early Mennonite life. The first northward migration took one group of Mennonites from the Netherlands to the Danzig-Vistula region, then under the rule of Polish kings (Sawatzky 1971). Over two hundred years later, when the Lutheran Church imposed severe restrictions on further land purchases by Mennonites, many moved on to South Russia, where the Russian Colonial Law of 1763 offered them free land, "perpetual exemption from military and civil service, freedom of religion, the right to control their schools and churches, and the right (and obligation) of agricultural colonies to be locally autonomous" (Sawatzky 1971: 5).[4] After almost one hundred years of prosperous and self-governed colony life, the Russian tsar began to withdraw privileges of cultural-religious freedom and autonomy. Most importantly, military exemption was no longer permitted, as the Mennonites were required to fulfill all responsibilities as Russian citizens. The majority of Mennonites agreed to render some form of service to the state, while others understood the compromises demanded by the tsar to be irreconcilable with Mennonite beliefs and practices.

Ideological dissension within the Mennonite brotherhood, coupled with intensifying problems of landlessness and inadequate alternative economic opportunities, enticed many to look to a new land. Between 1874 and 1880, over one third of the fifty thousand Mennonites in Russia immigrated to North America. Most settled in southern Manitoba, where the Canadian government offered inexpensive land to establish their closed colonies. But less than a decade later, the provincial government instituted the Manitoba Schools Act that required all instruction to be in English, and later stipulated that all public schools fly the Union Jack. Internal conflict among the Mennonites again flared. Some began moving west, and by 1911, the Canadian census reported 14,400 Mennonites in Saskatchewan and 15,600 in Manitoba (Sawatzky 1971: 18). When both the Manitoba and Saskatchewan governments implemented the School Attendance Act in 1916 in an attempt to assimilate ethnic groups and eliminate the German language in all schools, Mennonites who did not send their children to a recognised English-speaking school were fined or incarcerated. With mounting pressures of World War I, military conscription was imposed in 1917.

Even under these extreme conditions, the more 'liberal' among the Mennonites continued to find ways to adjust to government demands; but the more conservative groups—the Old Colony (or *Altkolonier*) and *Sommerfelder*—became increasingly disturbed by the perceived threats to church authority and community cohesiveness, and seven thousand members emigrated once again, this time to Latin America (Epp 1982; Janzen 2004; Sawatzky 1971). This migration to Latin America distinguishes

Low German Mennonite groups, as I identify them, from the wide range of other Mennonite groups that remained settled after immigrating to Canada and the United States. As a result of growing concern among the Mennonite communities remaining in Canada about the possibility of mandated direct military involvement, a second wave of migrations to Paraguay and Mexico occurred when international travel was made possible following World War II, and more southern colonies were formed in the 1940s and 1950s. In the past eighty years, Mennonite colonies consisting of smaller units of numbered 'campos' have sought land for further settlement in the Mexican states of Chihuahua, Durango, Campeche, and Zacatecas.

Disillusioned by broken promises and economic hardship, the movement of Low German Mennonites back to Canada began as early as a decade after the first migrations south. Economic and social conditions have meant that survival within closed Mennonite colonies in Mexico and Bolivia has not been possible for everyone. Therefore, for Low German Mennonites, hope was invested in obtaining 'papers.' With documentation proving Canadian citizenship (by birth) for at least one adult family member, thousands of Low German Mennonites have left their communities in Latin America in the past four decades to try to 'make a living' in Canada.

Today, Low German Mennonites in Canada number an estimated fifty thousand to sixty thousand, most in areas close to the fertile farming fields of Ontario, Alberta, Saskatchewan, and Manitoba (Janzen 1998; Loewen 2007). Some continue to migrate between Canada and their colony to the south, finding employment on Canadian farms and returning south when the work runs out and winter sets in. Others attempt to 'settle' more permanently in Canada, making the long drive back to Mexico only for extended vacations in the winter months. And there are some for whom any chance of return, even for a visit with family, is financially and logistically impossible.

Transnational migration is clearly not new for Low German Mennonites. Indeed, some have argued that the Mennonite ethno-cultural and religious way of life gives expression to a theology—a belief *and* way of life—of migration (Guenther 2000). Yet economic migration, which defines the more recent migrations from Latin America to Canada, is unprecedented in Mennonite history. These migrations, referred to by some church leaders as an "uncontrolled migration," consist of unsanctioned, familial moves from Latin America to Canada, which sharply distinguish them from all other migrations in Mennonite history.


## IN-BETWEEN SACRED/SECULAR-SPACE

In Latin America, Low German Mennonites know an *integrated life*, as all aspects of daily living—including school, church, clothing, language, and work—are to be preserved, with little change, within the tight boundaries of the colony. The Mennonite way of life is best described as a faith tradition. Anabaptism, and the various streams of Mennonite religious faith that emerged from it through the centuries, is a faith rooted in tradition and history, expressed in a way of life; and it is also a tradition, a history, and a way of life that is grounded in faith or religious beliefs. This was demonstrated repeatedly in the interview conversations with Low German Mennonite women. Translation of concepts of 'faith' or 'belief' proved to be difficult, if not impossible, and attempts to inquire about such were often met with uncertain and brief responses. Most women, however, were very clear about the *'right way to live.'* Emphasis is placed on obedience to acceptable practices and behaviour, rather than private, individual beliefs. In this way, faith must be publicly demonstrated.

Work is a cornerstone of the Mennonite faith tradition, because work is vital for preserving the right way of living. For Low German Mennonites, living *'so that God will be satisfied'* or so as to be a *'good church person'* is to work on the land. This esteemed life is one of subsistence farming, whereby the family functions as an economic unit. Even though gender roles are usually clearly defined, the division of labour between men and women is somewhat blurred, as every member of the family contributes to daily survival and all work is valued for its part towards the continuance of their way of life. Thus, Low German people describe working until there is enough. Many Mennonite (im)migrants seem indifferent to improving their position in the Canadian labour force or aspiring to 'make something of themselves.' For example, Jacob and Susana,[5] parents of fourteen children, described their hopes for their family, whether in Mexico or Canada:

Jacob.   [Trans.] [6] *I would wish that we could work as much that we could live good. Not overly enough, I wouldn't wish.*

Susana.   *Not that we had overly enough. That I wouldn't wish. Just so we always had enough to live.*

Low German Mennonite women know a separated life. Anabaptist/Mennonite peoples have historically defined themselves to be a people set apart. As distinct communities, Mennonites strive to be on the outside, segregated, distinct, and counter-cultural. The New Testament teaching to be *'in the world, but not of the world'*[7] demands a different way—a way of peace, of community, of simple living. To resist the world is *'to stay with what we have been taught.'* For all traditional Mennonite groups, including the Old Colony, faithfulness requires strict adherence to tradition and heritage. Change—to *'go beyond what I was taught'*—is to go the way of the world.

> *It seems to me, how would you say it, everything is advancing. In the last ten years how it's changed with all those cell phones and everything, so much new stuff. And the Dietsch, the children too, they go and get exactly the same things that everyone else has. They have everything—Internet, computers—and they're eager to get it. We*

*were always taught that we should not do as the world, we shouldn't have all that. We're supposed to stay away from what the world has. Of course the world will entice us, but we don't have to have it all. We shouldn't spend money on what isn't necessary.*

While non-conformity to the ways of the world is necessary for acceptance before God and church leaders, so too is conformity to the ways of the colony (Fast 2004). The communal or collective life is deeply rooted in Mennonite heritage. Low German colonies in Mexico were first established in accordance with the principles of equality and mutuality, as each family received the same amount of land to farm, and the cattle-grazing land was common to all. The tradition holds that to be Mennonite is to be part of the community, a faith community. This ideal is expressed as *Jemeenschauft*,[8] the everyday yet deeply spiritual quality of family and community relationships that is fundamental to the Mennonite faith tradition. One's consciousness, self-esteem, and whole sense of self are collective. The community defines the individual, and the individual belongs to the community, as the church seeks to be "of one heart and one soul" (Wiebe 1981: 33). This collective or shared self-esteem has to do with staying separate and different from the world, with more emphasis on eternity than the present. "*We were taught that the world is not going where we are going.*"

Further, to be a part of the community, the church, is to yield—to submit—to higher authorities: the will of God, the church, elders, parents, the community, and tradition. One Mennonite author describes this collective identity and yielding as "a master cultural disposition, deeply bred in the Mennonite soul, that governs perceptions, emotions, behaviour, and architecture" (Kraybill 2001: 30). The roots of this way of thinking can be traced to the Anabaptists of the sixteenth century, who believed that a dedicated heart would "forsake all selfishness," and "Christ called them to abandon self-interest and follow his example of suffering, meekness, humility, and service" (Kraybill 2001: 30). Such selflessness requires that individuals do not strive to stand out, or think independently, or be their own person. Rather, the best is to blend, to conform, and to submit to the group. Ideals of individual rights, freedoms, and choice are not only foreign to this way of thinking; they pose a threat. The needs of the group are always considered above the needs of any one of its members.[9] Low German women reported that many adults never dare to think or make decisions for themselves, as it is better to simply abide by the conventions and rules established by those in positions of higher authority.

Yielding to higher authorities means that one accepts what life brings. And life is suffering. An identity as a persecuted people seems to be genetically inscribed. All groups deriving from the Anabaptist martyrs know this identity. A certain virtue is associated with suffering, as the "pilgrim people of God" of all times have had to suffer "for living a non-conformed life of discipleship" (Guenther 2000: 169). Echoing the songs and poetry of the Old Testament, lamentations of persecution and hardship are often centrally represented in Mennonite music and literature.[10] This is in keeping with the values of self-denial, self-sacrifice, and selflessness. Resignation to the realities of life may mean tolerating conditions or illness—especially mental health or emotional difficulties—that can sometimes be ameliorated or treated. Righteousness dwells in the contrite heart, the yielding spirit.

Submission and collective identity are demonstrated most clearly by Low German Mennonite women. A woman knows herself as wife and mother, and her identity is firmly rooted in the family. A woman usually identifies herself by her husband's name, according to her family relationships. Furthermore, the work of a woman, her role in life—to further the church—defines her. She may occupy a position subordinate to her husband and to God, but she is vital to the preservation of her people. Tina Fehr Kehler (2004) writes this about Low German women from Mexico:

> [They] come from sacred villages—communities that are organized vis-à-vis the church. In Mexico, their life's work was geared to maintaining the church, community; that is raising children, baking bread and growing a garden were important though unrecognized ways in which the community of faith survived. Though women's work in Canada is no longer conducted in and for this sacred village, they continue to prepare the next generation for entry into the larger church. (22)

Many Low German Mennonite women demonstrated that their children and their role as mother are paramount for them. Preservation of religious tradition depends on women's work of reproduction—cultural, social, religious, and ethnic. A Low German Mennonite woman knows that her primary responsibility in life is to 'raise her children right.' Virtually every aspect of life (health care, housing, work, language) relates to caring work, raising children in the ways of their people. In this way, women's reproductive work is also fundamentally—and necessarily—material. This is God-ordained work with which they have been entrusted. To separate her from her family, the church, her people, is to strip her of her identity, of her self. It is to annihilate her.

Material hardship and socio-economic divides have eroded this integrated, separated, and collective life. Some families are forced into in-between places and spaces that are characterised by contradiction, confrontation, and conflict.

## CONTRADICTION OF IN-BETWEEN

Outside of the security and restrictions of colony life, migration is marked by contradiction. It is common in studies of migration to consider the 'push' and 'pull' factors that propel people out of place. Most often, these terms refer to socio-economic conditions in countries of origin, and international trade and labour agreements with destination countries. The push factors for most Mennonites from Mexico are profoundly commonplace, as they are experienced by millions of people all over the world. At least five inter-related factors are presented in the data:

- Economic restructuring in Mexico resulting from neoliberal policies, so that employment is extremely scarce, and small farmers incur rising expenses while earning dramatically declining incomes from their products
- Extreme climate conditions—drought alternating with flooding—resulting in poor crop yields year after year
- Growing pressures on the land base, so that young married couples often have no way of providing for a family within the colony
- Escalating violence and 'lawlessness'[11]
- Personal financial destitution and debt

Together, these intensifying conditions result in severe material hardship and widening social and economic divides, as also seen within and between societies all across the globe. The gap between rich and poor has permeated many of the Mennonite colonies in Latin America: large and lucrative farms sit alongside dilapidated shacks. Wealth and poverty are uncommonly close neighbours, contributing to conflict, corruption, and violence—even within colonies and families.[12]

In the contradictory spaces of social divides, cultural and religious life is threatened, and the borders shielding the sacred from the secular cannot be secured. In Latin America, a great deal of effort is invested in protecting church members within the sanctuary of the colony, so that when Low German Mennonites are confronted with desperate economic conditions, impossible choices must be made.

*Helena.*   [Trans.] *And it is too that there is more work here* [Canada]. *There, there isn't as much work as here. There they have to drive out to places, and that's what we didn't want. We didn't want our people in amongst the Mexicans. That's why we came here. There's more work here. . . . Many people, they just have the place with the house, and they just have to go to work.*

*Translator.*   [Trans.] *Do they have to go to a Mexican town to find work?*

*Helena.*   [Trans.] *Yeah, many do. And it isn't their freedom, from our leaders. It is not allowed, but they finally can't do it. Everything is full. Acreage land, and the cheese factories, and stores, shops—that's all full. It's all full of workers. And then besides, there are many places where they don't have room* [on the land].

> *They have to find a way of making a living, and then have to go to see what to find. My husband has long years worked with pumps, with well drills.*

Translator.    [Trans.] *And that was with Mexicans?*

Helena.    [Trans.] *Always drove out. He didn't have anything else. There in the colony, there wasn't room. No work. And he'd drive out Monday morning and come back Saturday, and he worked with the wells for the Mexicans.*

Luann.    *But it was not endorsed by the church leaders to go and work outside of the community.*

Helena.    [Trans.] *Rightly said. We did not have the freedom, but since it was all full and not enough work for everyone, they have to let them go and find work.*

In Mexico, urgency accompanies this ancestral and collective disposition as 'foreigner' in one's own country.

> [Trans.] *In Mexico, there are many villages, many villages. You can go from one to the other, go from one to the other, with horse and buggy. But we can keep the kids in the village. Yes, there's a lot of noise, shouting, they're often loud. But they're all Dietsch, all Dietsch. Nobody else has to get into a knot about it. They're all "us."*

Low German respondents expressed grave concern—even fear—for their young people, as they are increasingly engaged with Mexican society—a society generally held responsible for the growing drug and alcohol problem among Low German Mennonites (Castro 2004). Continuing the pattern of their migratory history, some families look towards a new land when worldliness begins to penetrate the borders of the colony. Individual migration—unsanctioned by the church and thus a denunciation of religious ideals—ironically also constitutes an act of religious steadfastness, as it gives expression to their traditional inclination towards preservation of separation and distinction from the world around.

Physical survival is also threatened by deepening socio-economic divides. Migration is necessity for many—a pragmatic decision that is both cause and consequence of cultural and religious alienation. Most women who have migrated to Canada reported that there was simply no way for them to make a living inside or outside the colony.

> [Trans.] *There, it wasn't possible for husbands to get employment. They were at home, but there wasn't enough work for them to do. So what were they supposed to do? They went to town, drank, and the wife with her small children sat at home and cried. She didn't know where her husband was. Her husband got bored at home, didn't know what to do with himself because there was no work. There wasn't*

*enough land, there wasn't enough for them to do and they got bored. Neither did they have money. If he wanted to work at something, fix the fence or build a shed, or a new house, create work for themselves, there was never money to do it. So the little bit of money he had, he could go to town and sit in bars and drink. His wife with her little kids, sat at home and cried. She waited, it got dark, night time came, and he didn't come. She didn't know if he was still alive or what he was up to.*

Many families sell everything to finance their move, and some accrue enormous debt in order to migrate north. The day-to-day struggle for physical survival sometimes leads to despair, and some who migrate have given up the dream of an agrarian way of life.

Luann.  *And what would allow people to make that decision, to take that step?*

Nancy.  *Desperation, I think. When a person gets desperate, he will break rules, he will break laws, you know. And I think that's the biggest thing. For people that are desperate to survive, or that are desperate to . . . do something different or better. I think desperation.* [Low German Mennonite service provider]

In addition to the cogent 'push' factors, the 'pull' to Canada is increasingly apparent. The growing demand for cheap labour in the North has given rise to expanding avenues for migration—authorised and unauthorised— for workers made poor in the South (Good Gingrich 2010). For Low German Mennonites, migratory pathways between Latin America and Canada have been facilitated by the possibility of Canadian citizenship, as familial connections with Canada are several generations old. For some, migration affords family reunification. In contrast, some families are painfully divided by geography, citizenship, religious disagreement, and sometimes financial disputes.

In Canada, where the colony way of life has been left behind, many seek agricultural employment opportunities that offer housing on the employing farm property. The work that is preferred is close to home, in the fields, so that families can work together to make a living.[13] In this way, the most highly valued work is domestic, in the sense that the boundaries between home, church, and community are permeable and largely undifferentiated. Providing for one's family and furthering the church are both realised primarily through work. It is right and good that the whole family works together towards their livelihood. When necessary, children go to work in the fields to help boost the family's income. When possible, the young women and girls in the family work inside the home, learning the skills of mothering and homemaking. Boys work outside, with their fathers, learning to live from and with the land. In Canada as in Latin America, church, community, family, faith, language, culture, and ethnicity are all protected as one. The Low German way of life, in place and space in-between, is political, as it sharply contradicts and thus challenges the values and beliefs of the dominant, secular world around them.


## CONFRONTATION OF IN-BETWEEN

Without the material resources necessary to establish themselves as autonomous, self-sufficient—and therefore 'integrated'—citizens promptly upon their arrival, most Mennonite (im)migrants from Latin America find themselves necessarily engaged with local social services. Ironically, it is when women and children encounter the social worker that Low German families are confronted with the full force of the market.

For many Mennonite families, considerable need follows them from the South to the North. This is disturbing for service providers in Canada, because need signifies *risk* in our marketised social policy and social service systems (Swift and Callahan 2009). In Canada, Mennonite (im)migrant women and their children in particular are understood to be vulnerable to the "moral hazards" of the welfare state (Martin 2004, 2010) due to a whole host of social and personal threats to their individual independence. Service providers find most aspects of their daily practices and cultural-religious norms to be problematic, interrelated, and 'compounding,' in that it was not possible to name issues of concern as discrete and disconnected from each other. For example, their large families, migration habits, poor language skills, work preferences, and low levels of education are all seen by service providers to contribute to difficulties for Mennonites in obtaining adequate and affordable housing, steady employment and sufficient income, education for their children, good health care, and social supports. Their strong commitment to family networks and traditional gender roles is assumed to translate into tolerance for, or even endorsement of, harsh domination of women and children. Almost always, Mennonites prefer to live 'in the country,' where affordable and adequate housing is quite scarce. It is common for families to live in tobacco houses, chicken coops, bunk houses, and house trailers. When the family has only one vehicle, as is often the case, many women lack any means of transportation, and remain quite isolated in their own homes. Often, *Plautdietsch* (Low German) is spoken in the workplace as well as the home. With little opportunity or occasion to leave the family home, many women have very poor English-language skills, even years after settling in Canada. Service providers observed that many attend their own churches, prefer their own schools (if they send children to school at all), and attempt to stay "*totally separate like a colony in Mexico.*"

Defining social problems is complicated work in the "social problems industry" (Loseke 2003). Social service workers seldom agree on what is wrong, much less how to make it right. This is apparent in the widely divergent—even contradictory—assessments by Canadian service providers of the economic and social circumstances of Low German families. Most service providers readily acknowledged the desperate conditions that many Mennonites left behind in Latin America. Some postulate that the Low German population represents an unusually impoverished group of immigrants:

> *When they come from Mexico, there is nothing there. They come from very, very poor villages and there is nothing! And it—well, a doctor called me once because he was sending a woman home having had a baby and he said, "Is the environment suitable?" I said, "Well, no. For you, no. You wouldn't consider it suitable, but for what they're used to, this is heaven. Like, they have floors; they have doors!"* [English service provider]

It is recognised that even in Canada, some Mennonite (im)migrants have difficulty providing the basic necessities for their families:

> *When we go into families, we can have a gamut of abuse sometimes— physical abuse, and parent-teen conflict, children's behaviour being out of control, mom not able to cope if dad's not in the home. But we find we can't even address those things until we actually address the level of poverty some of them are living in. It just blows some of my staff away. I mean, you can't work on anything around parenting skills, or setting up structure, or routine in the home without first addressing, "When am I going to get food to feed my children tomorrow?" So we find that is a real core issue with quite a few families that we have.* [English service provider]

On the other hand, some practitioners commented on the extraordinary potential for earnings in a single picking season when several family members contribute. One social service worker speculated that a family working together in tomato or cucumber fields could make *"over ten thousand dollars in one month."* This in combination with the Child Tax Benefit[14] money collected by many of these large families led some service providers to wonder what some families do with their money—that perhaps they are *"hiding what they have in bank accounts,"* buying properties for their sons, contributing large sums of money to the church or extended family members, or simply squandering their earnings.

While social service workers did not agree on the identification or prioritization of problems among Low German families, the thrust of interventions was articulated with noticeable consistency and resolve. Staff from employment programmes, social services, school boards, public health, mental health, and primary health care agreed that a principal goal of their work is to help people—men and women alike—get and keep a job. This is accomplished primarily through providing specific training and education programmes for client groups, with a view towards encouraging their appropriate participation in the labour market and society in general. The issue is not that Mennonite (im)migrants are considered lazy or unmotivated, or even unproductive.

> *I'd say one of their strengths too is their work ethic. It's very, very strong, and they're not afraid of physical labour, and menial labour. You know, they never shy away from any type of work. They'll work the long hours, the overtime.* [English service provider]

Rather, employment, housing, language, education, size of families, and migration patterns form a single, coherent risk that translates into objectionable participation in the labour force. The priority, for many service providers, is to discourage the Low German preference for field work.

Mike.    *Some of the mothers have taken their children and are trying to forge a new life for them.*
Louise.   *It's a lonely life.*
Mike.    *Yeah, but I mean, in this one case, the two daughters, the mother made sure they completed their high school. One's going on to post secondary. One's working at Wendy's. At least it's not working in the fields, you know.* [English service providers]

Employment-oriented social welfare services, such as the workfare programmes that have replaced welfare in most of North America, base eligibility for benefits on some form of labour market engagement. Confronted with the limited options of an increasingly polarised labour market, social workers are routinely required to redirect their clients into equally low-paying jobs with poor working conditions in precarious sectors of the labour market. Marketised social services present dilemmas and paradox for workers and recipients alike.

Market logic conflates paid work with financial security, recognition, social legitimacy and inclusion, and personal liberation—especially for women. Making a living is reduced to earning a wage. But the everyday realities of immigrant women's lives do not support such blind faith. It is here, at this point, that conflict occurs—when Low German Mennonite women are deemed lacking, and social workers and health providers seek to improve life for Mennonite women and children. It is conflict provoked by confrontation between competing ideals and aspirations, and even more, contradictory livelihood practices and sensibilities in the everyday.

## CONFLICT OF IN-BETWEEN

According to market logic, all value is associated with individual bodily expressions of autonomy, competition, choice, self-sufficiency, precise whiteness, and heterosexual maleness. In marketised social services, the ideal *client* subject stands for lack, and provides a negative comparator for the ideal *citizen* subject.[15]

The ethnocentrism and individualism of economism in the delivery of social services acknowledge and permit only competitive self-interest and exchanges, disallowing and vilifying any evidence of a cooperative "good-faith economy" (Bourdieu 1990: 115). Such personal transactions and communal relationships, common among the Low German Mennonites, are considered suspect and even fraudulent if conducted by social service clients. Social service workers reported that Mennonite service recipients are penalised for 'pooling family resources,' or accepting monetary gifts or loans. Thus, any material or social cushion afforded by the remaining remnants of the Mennonite collective lifestyle is subverted. The more dispossession marks a person, the greater the potency of the forces that divide and isolate.

Field work and caring work are afforded little worth in the singular system of capital—the rules of the game—that organises the social welfare system and the market. Employment as a farm labourer is usually seasonal, unregulated, and low paying. Caring labour, when conducted in one's own home for family members, is made invisible and inconsequential. In market terms, such activity is not counted as work at all. Prince (2001) argues, "The guiding principle for reforming social programs is that they support the work ethic and economic productivity" (6). Market morality serves to define and valuate all things in its own terms. Thus, in the marketised social services system, the value of women's work and its contribution to the livelihood of the family is discounted, reduced to the wages her labour earns.

*Jen.*     *We probably should tell them about our sewing project.*

*Kathleen. Oh yeah. That's a good one.*

*Jen.*     *We have fifty Low German women sewing out of their own homes for a company in London. And that was a big project that we just got . . .*

*Kathleen. A very high percentage of those women had never worked outside of the home.*

*Jen.*     *They've never worked outside of the home. Most of them with grade four education.*

*Kathleen. And they have several of these sewing things, and these ladies are providing the best quality in . . .*

*Jen.*     *The company is really happy with them.*

*Kathleen. . . . the whole company.*

*Luann. Is this for hospital garb?*

*Jen.*     *Sewing scrubs. All the pieces are delivered to them. They just pick them up, and then they bring their finished product back. They're making some money and they're right in their own home, and . . .*

*Kathleen.* They can still meet the obligations of their homes. That's right. That's so empowering to be earning money, and . . .

*Jen.* The company got them their machines, and what they're doing is taking the cost of the machines as payroll deductions. So they had to sign a form just saying they would pay back, I forget—it was twenty-five dollars a pay, or twenty dollars a pay, or something until the machine is paid for. Some even opted to get a better quality machine, because they felt even if this job came to an end they would still use the machine. A lot of them sew their own children's clothing, and that kind of thing.

*Kathleen.* And the word is spreading! It's really . . .

*Jen.* It's spreading. We have a list of about sixty-five women that have signed on to try doing it once we need more.

*Kathleen.* We had started with using anybody who was interested, and all of the Canadian people dropped out. They didn't work out at all!

*Jen.* These Low German women are so committed, though. If they say are going to do twenty-five hours a week, they will do twenty-five hours a week. Even if they are in their own home. Where some others may say they will do twenty-five, and do five.

*Kathleen.* Or say, "This isn't worth it." But that's because you have other options. For these ladies there isn't another option, so they're saying, "Oh this is great." So, they're doing it. [English service providers]

Even more, Mennonite traditional labour of making a living is associated with illegitimacy and devaluation. Particularly when children help in the fields, seasonal workers may be paid in cash, 'under the table.' Situated in the 'informal economy' and shared by all family members, such work then takes on an illicit quality. Similarly, women's traditional work is disallowed for social service clients, as only waged work—although intensely precarious, low-wage, unregulated, and dead-end—counts for anything at all. Mennonite (im)migrant women's roles and identities are not only cheapened; they are made dishonourable and ultimately costly. Such expressions of 'proximity to necessity' (Bourdieu 1984) mark Low German women as unworthy, and justify the denial of all possibility for social and even economic gain in both the social service system and the labour market. In this way, the livelihood strategies of Low German Mennonite women function in reverse, earning negative social and economic returns in all social arenas of Canadian society in which they must engage.

The Low German Mennonite collective sense of self—sometimes described by service providers as arrogance and even racism—poses a direct challenge to the neoliberal individual as a self-contained unit. Nancy, who is both a service provider and a member of the Low German community, looked for English words to describe this inclination towards denial of self, and she rather awkwardly settled on the familiar notion of 'poor self-esteem.'

Luann.   *I want to back up to your concern of "poor self-esteem," because that's something I've heard from others. How common is that among . . .*

Nancy.   *Very, very common. I mean, I think it's one of the biggest problems in our Mennonite community. It's a teaching also. From where I stand now, looking back, it's actually a teaching. You don't think much of yourself. If you were to think of yourself that you're able to do things, well, that's not right. We are being taught not to brag about ourselves. Not to think of ourselves as someone. Just simply not to think that you're somebody, you know. That would be the plainest way of explaining it. I mean, if . . . Parents are not encouraged to motivate their children, or to say, "You did really good." Because they may become too proud.*

Luann.   *So if you can think poorly of yourself, there's almost something righteous about that.*

Nancy.   *Right. Exactly.*

In the conflict of in-between, all strength afforded through the dialectical social individual—the self-in-community—is reversed, converted to an internalised sense of individual worthlessness and even self-contempt.

Low German and English workers alike described wasted potential in Low German young people, as they are often not encouraged to imagine beyond traditional livelihood strategies and roles. Service providers attributed such values, goals, and aspirations in Low German children and young people to parenting inadequacies and incompetence. Education through the public school system, employment services, custom-designed language and health programmes, individual instruction by a range of professionals and paraprofessionals, and even educational spots delivered over the waves of the Low German radio station are all geared towards encouraging or forcing changes in the way Low German Mennonites raise their children.

Through education—the most urgent need and preferred intervention strategy identified by service providers—workers seek to "shape minds and mould desires from within" (Wacquant 1996: 161). By way of education, training, assessing, and monitoring, social services work together towards the same end—producing compliance and conformity. Low German mothers must display a submissive confidence that 'worldly' interventions into the lives of their families are good and necessary, and must perform an ignorant belief that 'English' professionals know what is best for them and their children. Enforced compliance and conformity reinforce lack and dependency. This is the ideal client subject, and it serves to sustain the myth of the opposite kind. The standard of the 'self-made man' and the idealisation of individualised success can be preserved only through the manufacture of dispossessed social groups and their individualised failure. Clients must demonstrate independent and personal destitution—the complete absence of resources from family or community members—to establish legitimate need. The eligible client is necessarily made individualised, commodified, conformed, and compliant—giving rise to double binds of all sorts for Mennonite (im)migrant women.

## DOUBLE BINDS OF IN-BETWEEN

The Mennonite fundamental of an integrated, separated, and collective life is both undermined and intensified in migration. For example, living in closed communities in close geographic proximity is not possible in Canada, and categorical divisions between home and school and church and work come to define daily life. No longer bound by the rigid rules of the church, women (and men) have to make life decisions independent of family networks and religious authorities. Geographical, emotional, and religious separation from extended family and the church contribute to new forms of isolation for women in Canada. Women are required to conform to the ways of the world: discard her traditional dress and language, learn to read and write, find paid work, and leave her children to the secular education system. By *'working out,'* women are challenging religious definitions of what it is to be a good mother and wife. For Mennonite (im)migrant women, the peril associated with education and knowledge goes beyond worldly change and infiltration from the outside; the danger coupled with 'standing out,' being different, is rejection and expulsion from within, as it unsettles the God-ordained order of authority. Furthermore, the risks of women losing their children—to the child welfare system, or to the worldly ways of the ever-encroaching secular society—are great in Canada. And in Canada, where the borders of the colony no longer exist, men are free to come and go. Some husbands and fathers find the pressures of poverty and social exclusion to be unbearable, and they flee—sometimes taking refuge in a bottle, sometimes in the desperate familiarity of life in Mexico or Bolivia.

Yet, women expressed sincere gratitude for the abundance of their lives in Canada. Employment in farming fields, which is readily available during harvest seasons in rural Canada, offers an approximation of the agrarian life and work that represents hope (Kasdorf 1995). Even more, when confronted with the secular in migration, women's work takes on new meaning. Outside the structures of the colony, the family home rather than the church is the centre of economic, cultural, religious, and educational activity; and women become the 'keepers of the faith.' In spaces *entredeux*, women's work is the essence of their very survival.

The devalued necessity of women's work is central to the paradox of transnational livelihoods for Low German Mennonite women. I suggest that when we consider the ways in which transnational livelihoods impact women's households, it becomes apparent that this paradox is more than a sort of contradiction in terms—it is conflict, strife, brought on by all sorts of double binds in places and spaces in-between. Work sustains and divides; life outside the colony isolates and connects; new freedom is opportunity and burden; laws protect individual women and children, and threaten collective family life; waged work offers some economic liberation for women, and compromises and devalues their traditional roles and identities; and ultimately, migration preserves and destroys (Good Gingrich and Preibisch 2010). To migrate is to turn one's back on a tradition, on a heritage, on a life that has let you down.

> [Trans.] *Right way, we got married, had children. We were taught that we should have children, and we shouldn't use birth control* [literally: use something for it] *because they were a gift from God. That's what we wanted. But there wasn't land. Why didn't they* [church leadership] *prepare for it so that their people could stay there?*

And migration severs relationships with the living and the dead. Migration is an act of self-betrayal.

> [Trans.] *I moved away from my parents, I didn't have any family here* [in Canada]. *Later one of my sisters moved here as well. My mother cried a lot, "My children are gone, are gone. They are living where they aren't supposed to." My sister felt bad about my mother. But what are you supposed to do? My parents were perhaps two, three years old when they moved from Saskatchewan to Mexico. They taught us that we weren't supposed to return; they had removed us from there and we weren't supposed to return. But because there wasn't land—people just didn't have land—there wasn't work. So people were returning anyway. And we often feel bad about that. Mostly, we worry about that. We didn't obey. We didn't do as they taught us, but we had to! We also wanted to provide for our family. Our parents died long ago. Did we do right? They told us not to, but we did. It's confusing, isn't it?*

Caught in the contest between physical and cultural/religious survival, women find themselves in spaces *entredeux*—in-between tradition and rapid change, steadfastness and destabilisation, desperation and excess. For Mennonite (im)migrant women, transnational livelihoods require navigating necessity and absurdity, hope and hopelessness, faithfulness and condemnation. In this context of market neo-liberalism, in which choice and self-determination and individual autonomy are at once a unified ideal and illusion, the double bind of transnational livelihoods is the day-to-day reality of having no choice in every act of choosing (Good Gingrich and Preibisch 2010). To be forced to choose without really choosing—over and over—is to vacillate between, always in-between, colony life and the transnational life, in-between migration and settlement. It is to be caught in the nothing of *entredeux*, to be nowhere.

## A STORY OF IN-BETWEEN

The everyday realities of these conflicted places and spaces in which women live are best illustrated through a story—a true story, of a Low German Mennonite woman. Sarah came to Canada with her husband and their two young children over ten years ago. They left their colony in Mexico to find work. Land in their colony was scarce, and very expensive. Their extended families were poor, and didn't own enough land to provide for the families of their many children. Sarah and her husband couldn't afford to buy a house, much less enough land to sustain themselves. Her husband could find only short-term, poorly paid jobs outside of the colony, and their parents were continually critical of him mixing with Mexicans. It seemed there was no hope for them there. So they migrated to Canada, hoping to earn enough money to some day return to a Mennonite colony and begin their life together again. For the first three years or so, Sarah, her husband, and often their young children worked together in the cucumber and tomato fields in Ontario. The money was good during the harvest season, and there was always plenty of work. But after five years in Canada, their dream of colony life seemed dim.

Sarah had become a cooperative and eager social services client and student. She made the most of the services that were provided to her. With the help of social workers and health professionals, she was able to make significant changes in her life since arriving in Canada. She was no longer helping her husband in the fields. Instead, three days a week she attended an English-language programme for Low German women, and in this way met the job preparation requirements of the local workfare programme so that she could collect a monthly welfare cheque. She learned to speak English well enough to communicate with cashiers in the grocery store and even teachers at school. She was learning to read, for the first time in her life. She was receptive to information and advice about birth control, and made the unusual decision to have only three children. While she continued to wear a skirt and a head covering, she stopped sewing traditional dresses for herself. As her children reached school age, she kept the attendance counsellor at bay by ensuring that they regularly attended the local public school—even when the cruelty of other children left them fearful, begging to stay home. And most importantly, she left her controlling and abusive husband, and made a home for herself and her children.

I met Sarah when I was visiting this English-language programme for Low German Mennonite women in preparation for conducting my research. In her high-heeled boots, jean skirt, and long hair left flowing down her back, her appearance was more similar to the English teachers and staff than the Low German Mennonite students. My role that day was to teach a class on child nutrition, and I needed a translator. Sarah was a somewhat shy but willing volunteer. It was clear that her language skills were well beyond most of the other women attending the programme. She approached me after the class, an extraordinarily daring gesture for a Low German woman, and we chatted.

I was interested in interviewing Sarah for my research, because she seemed to be such an unusual woman in her community. When I asked about her at the end of the day, I learned that, like most Low German women who leave their husbands, she had become an outcast among her own people. Women and men alike refused to speak with her. Especially among more traditional groups, men regard single women to be available. When she feared for her own safety and the safety of her children, she had gone into hiding. She moved. She changed and unlisted her phone number. The teachers and social workers at the programme were pleased, however, as she and her children seemed to be managing quite well. With the occasional use of the food bank, she was able to get by on welfare. She was appearing more self-assured, making good decisions, acquiring new skills and knowledge, and demonstrating increasing independence. In contrast to many Old Colony Mennonite women around her, she was doing everything 'right.'

I returned a few months later, ready to begin my research. When I asked if Sarah might be contacted to request her participation in my study, I was told that she had disappeared. No one had heard anything from her for several weeks. Her regular attendance at English-language classes had suddenly stopped, which triggered cancellation of her social assistance cheques, her only source of income. Without warning or explanation, her children were no longer attending school. Several years later, there is still no word from Sarah. The social service workers who knew her best assumed that she returned to Mexico, to colony life, to desperate poverty, to the security of her extended family, to corruption and seeming lawlessness, to the life she believes to be faithful, and to her abusive husband.

## CONCLUSIONS AND IMPLICATIONS

Market-based welfare programmes, now commonplace in developed capitalist societies all over the world (OECD 2005), aim to increase economic self-reliance by redirecting people towards paid work and market consumption, and away from state-funded social services and assistance. Policy and programme measures include curtailing benefits, tightening eligibility, mandating employment-related activities, and punishing recipients for non-compliance (Lightman, Mitchell, and Herd 2010; Martin 2010). These 'reforms' work to channel all goals and means of benefits and services through paid market employment, and treat all social services as market-place commodities. This unqualified and exclusive alignment with the ethic of the economic market gives expression to a significant international ideological shift of welfare states over the past four decades. I argue that this represents more than a collaboration or partnership between the state and the market—it constitutes a corporate takeover of sorts, whereby the welfare state has been bought out by global market interests, thus imposing the market as the only game in town.

This market-state merger renders welfare policies and practices rife with contradiction. For example, Canada's social policies and related interventions and programmes—while they may be relatively generous and well-intentioned—operate to keep people—down-groups *and* up-groups—in place. The "possessive individualism" (Macpherson 1962) of the market-state, and all its associated hyper-valorisations, is fundamentally dependent—ironically so—on the production of various versions of 'dispossessed individualism.' The (im)migrant woman and her children are especially suitable for this enterprise, as her difference is seldom perceived to be strength or capacity; rather, difference is readily assessed to be lack. Her eligibility for the beleaguered and often punitive services of the market-state is evaluated monthly, and she is repeatedly made deficient and devalued. Furthermore, traditional women's work—in the home and in the fields—is made illicit for the dispossessed in the market-state. She is thus denied the strategies and roles and identities she knows to make a life, against all odds, and her dependency on the market is enforced. Even more, marketised social services paradoxically operate to augment need or lack that is reduced to the individual failure. For example, it was evidenced that processes and practices of Canada's marketised social services operate to further dispossess and devalue (im)migrant women who are marginal in the Low German community—women who are deficient and deviant according to their own cultural-religious rules for who gets ahead and who falls behind—in informal *and* formal systems of social support. Their material, social, and emotional suffering is intensified through voluntary or mandated engagement with a social services system that functions to sustain opposite social kinds and positions, thus deepening economic, social, and subjective divides.

For millions of people on the move, migration across national borders is survival. People are thrust into spaces in-between that are not easily escaped, even in wealthy welfare states of the world. The everyday realities of women reveal the ways in which gendered (and racialised) processes and structures are crucial in the production and reproduction of market-state social relations.[16] Particularly for groups seeking to preserve traditional cultural and religious practices in transnational spaces, daily life choices are complicated by pressures to conform to conflicting social fields.[17] The lives of Sarah and other Mennonite (im)migrant women provoke important questions for our consideration. How might social service workers recognise and even encourage traditional roles and identities afforded women in families and communities—roles and identities that are both confining and shielding, suffocating and fulfilling? What alternative ways of thinking and doing are required in the design and delivery of social services to utilise informal social support systems, and build on the collective know-how and capacity of families and communities to fend off all forms of social exclusion? More broadly, what reforms to national and international social policies and programmes are needed to validate and promote practices, values, and ideals that mediate rather than reproduce the inevitable contradictions of the market, towards the reconciliation of social divides?

## ACKNOWLEDGEMENTS

The author gratefully acknowledges the expert assistance of my research associate Dr. Kerry Fast, who thoroughly reviewed and commented on previous drafts of this chapter, and continues to deepen my understanding of Low German Mennonite life through our ongoing work together.

## NOTES

1. I use the term (im)migrant throughout the chapter to signify the Low German Mennonite transnational or supra-national disposition. Their migratory history that many continue today, and general resistance to 'settlement,' sharply distinguishes them from more conventional immigrants.
2. This research includes three projects, all funded by the Social Sciences and Humanities Research Council (SSHRC) of Canada: Good Gingrich, L. (2006) *Contesting Social Exclusion: An Interrogation of Its Self-Imposed Expressions*, PhD diss., Faculty of Social Work, University of Toronto; *Rural Women Making Change*, University of Guelph, principal investigator B. Leach, co-investigator K. Preibisch; *Theorizing 'Choice' and Voluntary Social Exclusion: A Study of Transnational Livelihoods and Women from Mexico*, York University, principal investigator L. Good Gingrich, co-investigator K. Preibisch.
3. The migration histories that have resulted in distinct Mennonite groups are described below.
4. These provisions, known as the eternal *Privilegium*, permitted the development of administrative and agricultural techniques that have become central to Mennonite institutions and their economic and cultural life. The *Privilegium* became a standard set of conditions used in seeking a new homeland in future migrations (Epp 1974).
5. All names of research participants have been changed to preserve anonymity.
6. When the words were originally offered in Low German and simultaneously transcribed and translated into English, the text is preceded by the following bracketed information: [Trans.].

7. Although a number of passages in the New Testament refer to the idea of non-conformity to the ways of the world, Romans 12:2 is commonly cited.
8. The full meaning of the Low German word *Jemeenschauft* is not easily captured in a single English word. The notion of 'fellowship' comes close in its reference to a spiritual dimension of community relationships, to something greater than the 'everyday.' Yet in Low German, it is also an everyday word to describe meaningful interaction between people, such as a good visit with a friend. It signifies the quality of an interaction, and the connection enjoyed through relating with each other (Fast 2011).
9. In an interview for a previous study with Old Order Mennonite informal helpers, one respondent recalled his sense of alarm and foreboding when the Human Rights Act was introduced in Canada in 1985. He described the underlying difficulty in determining whose individual rights and freedoms take precedence when they are contradictory. For him, the common good must always supersede the rights of any one individual (Good Gingrich and Lightman 2004).
10. It is said that the only book cherished more by Mennonites than the Bible is *Martyrs' Mirror*. Indeed, this book occupies a prominent place in the libraries of many Mennonite homes and churches. Consisting of a rather gruesome and lengthy report, it details the martyred deaths of hundreds of Anabaptists in the sixteenth century.
11. Several Low German women described Mexico as a place of "lawlessness." In contrast, women expressed gratitude for a greater sense of safety in Canada due to laws that protect them and their children. It is not my intention to unfairly represent the state of law enforcement and social order in a diverse and evolving society. I use the term here to indicate what I understand to be the perception of many (im)migrants who have experienced violence inside or outside their colonies in Mexico.
12. Economic disparity within Mennonite colonies has resulted in part from the traditional system for allocating land that combines collectivism and shared ownership with market competition. For example, when a new colony was established, each family was provided with the same allotted number of hectares, each piece of land straddling the village street. Because the custom is to have a house for your child when he/she gets married, families built a second house, often on the other side of the street. Thus, each family's parcel of land had to support more people, and the number of dwellings in a village increased exponentially while the number of landowners declined. Over time, land has become very scarce—and therefore very expensive—on some of the more established colonies (such as those near Durango, Mexico, and Riva Palacios Colony in Bolivia). These colonies have become overcrowded; an increasingly small proportion of families owns colony land; more are tenants of—and indebted to—a few; and more are seeking employment within or outside of the colony. Desperation leads to migration for some, and disparity is exacerbated as only wealthier families are able to purchase more land for their children or for their own expansion when land becomes available (Fast 2011).
13. Even though in Canada families often live on the farms where they work, their living conditions sharply contradict the meaning and experience of colony life in Mexico. For example, nuclear families live geographically and symbolically isolated from extended families and the religious community. Further, the cultural-religious norm—even imperative—of owning your own land and being your own boss is little more than a 'broken dream' in rural Canada.

14. The federal Child Tax Benefit is a monthly, tax-free cash supplement calculated per child—paid to eligible low- and middle-income applicants with children under eighteen years—usually issued to mothers, provided they hold status as citizens, landed immigrants, or refugees. For large families, research respondents report that the monthly benefit can amount to over C$1,000.
15. Orloff (2005) describes the universal political subject—the seemingly ungendered ideological icon—produced in social policy and related services to be "rational, autonomous, unburdened by care, impervious to invasions of bodily integrity and therefore (heterosexual and) masculine" (219). He is a producing, consuming, tax-paying citizen. Similarly, the necessary backdrop for all "incomplete," excluded subjects of western welfare capitalism is described to be "the white, male, able-bodied, wage-earning subject," "the 'independent' figure able to claim and enact legal, political and social rights" (Clarke 2003: 211).
16. See also Good Gingrich (2010).
17. For an insightful and thorough consideration of the contradictions of individual agency within the Low German Mennonite culture, see Fast (2004). Through the use of a poignant case example of a Low German Mennonite woman, Fast clearly demonstrates that questions of choice and agency are often too simply and falsely understood in narrow, individualised terms, and equated with "self-determination." Although the focus of her work is on this seemingly peculiar traditional religious group and a social context that demands a high degree of conformity, I argue that her understanding of agency as taking place within the constraints of a life and community is equally applicable and accurate in a traditional religious society and contemporary 'secular' societies.

## BIBLIOGRAPHY

Bourdieu, P. (1984) *Distinction: A Social Critique of the Judgement of Taste*. Cambridge, MA: Harvard University Press.
Bourdieu, P. (1990) *The Logic of Practice*. Translated by R. Nice. Stanford, CA: Stanford University Press.
Castro, P. (2004) 'The 'Return' of the Mennonites from the Cuauhtémoc Region to Canada: A Perspective from Mexico.' *Journal of Mennonite Studies*, 22: 25–38.
Cixous, H., and M. Calle-Gruber (1997) *Hélène Cixous, Rootprints : Memory and Life Writing: London*. New York: Routledge.
Clarke, J. (2003) 'Turning Inside Out? Globalization, Neo-liberalism and Welfare States.' *Anthropologica*, 45(2): 201–22.
Epp, F. H. (1974) *Mennonites in Canada, 1786–1920: The History of a Separate People*. Toronto: Macmillan of Canada.
Epp, F. H. (1982) *Mennonites in Canada, 1920–1940: A People's Struggle for Survival*. Toronto: Macmillan of Canada.
Fast, K. (2004) 'Religion, Pain, and the Body: Agency in the Life of an Old Colony Mennonite Woman.' *Journal of Mennonite Studies*, 22: 103–29.
Fast, K. (2011a) Personal communication. Toronto, 23 January.
Fast, K. (2011b) Personal communication. Toronto, 18 March.
Fehr Kehler, T. (2004). 'A Kanadier Mennonite Woman's Experience.' *Women's Concerns Report*, March-April, No. 172. Winnipeg: Mennonite Central Committee—Committees on Women's Concerns.

Good Gingrich, L. (2010) 'The Symbolic Economy of Trans-border Governance: A Case Study of Subjective Exclusion and Migrant Women from Mexico.' *Refugee Survey Quarterly*, 29(1): 161–84.

Good Gingrich, L., and E. Lightman (2004) 'Mediating Communities and Cultures: A Case Study of Informal Helpers in an Old Order Mennonite Community.' *Families in Society*, 85(4): 511–520.

Good Gingrich, L., and K. Preibisch (2010) 'Migration as Preservation and Loss: The Paradox of Transnational Living for Low German Mennonite Women.' *Journal of Ethnic and Migration Studies*, 36(9): 1499–518.

Guenther, T. F. (2000) 'Theology of Migration: The *Ältesten* Reflect.' *Journal of Mennonite Studies*, 18: 164–76.

Janzen, W. (1998) *Build Up One Another: The Work of MCCO with the Mennonites from Mexico in Ontario 1977–1997.* Kitchener, Ontario: Mennonite Central Committee Ontario.

Janzen, W. (2004) 'Welcoming the Returning "Kanadier" Mennonites from Mexico.' *Journal of Mennonite Studies*, 22: 11–24.

Kasdorf, J. (1995) 'Work and Hope: An Anabaptist Adam.' *Mennonite Quarterly Review*, 69(2): 178–204.

Kraybill, D. B. (2001) *The Riddle of Amish Culture.* Revised ed. Baltimore, MD: John Hopkins University Press.

Lightman, E., A. Mitchell, and D. Herd (2010) 'Cycling On and Off Welfare in Canada.' *Journal of Social Policy*, 39(4): 523–42.

Loewen, R. (2007) 'To the Ends of the Earth: Low German Mennonites and Old Order Ways in the Americas.' Paper given at the "Amish in America" Conference, Elizabethtown, PA, 7–9 June 2007.

Loseke, D. R. (2003) *Thinking about Social Problems: An Introduction to Constructionist Perspectives (Social Problems and Social Issues).* 2nd ed. New York: Aldine de Gruyter.

Macpherson, C. B. (1962) *The Political Theory of Possessive Individualism.* Oxford: Oxford University Press.

Martin, S. (2004) 'Reconceptualising Social Exclusion: A Critical Response to the Neoliberal Welfare Reform Agenda and the Underclass Thesis.' *Australian Journal of Social Issues*, 39(1): 79–94.

Martin, S. (2010) 'Reconceptualising Young People's Engagement with Work and Welfare: Considering 'Choice''. Paper given at the XVII International Sociological Association World Congress of Sociology, Gothenburg, Sweden, 11–17 July 2010.

Orloff, A. S. (2005). 'Social Provision and Regulation: Theories of States, Social Policies, and Modernity.' In J. Adams, E. S. Clemens & A. Shola Orloff (Eds.), *Remaking Modernity: Politics, History, and Sociology* (pp. 190–224). Durham: Duke University Press.

Organization for Economic Cooperation and Development (OECD) (2005) Policy Brief: 'From Unemployment to Work.' http://www.oecd.org/dataoecd/44/23/35044016.pdf (accessed 28 October 2011).

Prince, M. J. (2001) 'How Social Is Social Policy? Fiscal and Market Discourse in North American Welfare States.' *Social Policy & Administration*, 35(1): 2–13.

Sawatzky, H. L. (1971) *They Sought a Country: Mennonite Colonization in Mexico.* Los Angeles, CA: University of California Press.

Smith, D. E. (1999) *Writing the Social: Critique, Theory, and Investigations.* Toronto: University of Toronto Press.

Swift, K. J., and M. Callahan (2009) *At Risk: Social Justice in Child Welfare and Other Human Services.* Toronto: University of Toronto Press.

Wacquant, L. (1996) 'Reading Bourdieu's "Capital".' *International Journal of Contemporary Sociology*, 33(2): 151–70.

Wiebe, G. (1981) *Causes and History of the Emigration of the Mennonites from Russia to America*. Translated by H. Janzen. Winnipeg: Manitoba Mennonite Historical Society. Original edition, Ursachen und Geschichte der Auswanderung der Mennoniten aus Russland nach Amerika, 1900.

# 7 Sisters in Struggle?
## Wars Between Daughters-in-law and Migrant Workers

*Frank T. Y. Wang and Chin-ju Lin*

## INTRODUCTION

One of the characteristics of welfare states in East Asian countries is the influence of Confucian culture (Lee and Ku 2007; Kwon 2005; Holliday 2000; Ku, 1995; Jones 1993). Caring for frail family members is considered to be a family responsibility under the influence of Confucianism, rather than a social issue to be dealt with by the state. By privatising caring responsibility for frail persons, social policies become subordinate to economic policies, which are aimed at economic development. Although Taiwan, South Korea, and Japan share the influence of Confucian teaching, what distinguishes Taiwan from South Korea and Japan in its response to the growing needs for care is its relatively unrestricted policy on semi-skilled migrant domestic care workers.[1] The care work for frail persons in Taiwan is mainly provided at home by daughters-in-law, the designated caregivers within the traditional family discourse. As the tradition of family care becomes more and more difficult to achieve, a new group of women is made available through the recently formed global care chain, namely migrant care workers. At the intersection of traditional culture and globalised organisation of care work, the number of Taiwanese families that include both daughters-in-law and migrant care workers has been increasing during the last two decades. This chapter investigates the experiences of such families, especially the conflicts, tension, and struggles between Taiwanese daughters-in-law and migrant care workers, how they re-arrange housework, and how they negotiate the tension and conflicts between them.

The chapter is composed of two parts. In the first part, we will set the context for understanding the wars waging between two women within the household. The daughter-in-law role is socially constructed through Confucian teachings on family ethics that function to minimise the role of the state and to relegate women to the role of family caregiver in Taiwan. Then, in order to maintain the cultural image of family care, the need for an affordable source of care labour has been increasing. Over the past fifteen years, migrant domestic workers have become the most popular choice. Thus, a new woman emerges in the picture of Taiwanese family, i.e., the migrant domestic worker. Migrant domestic workers are a result of the historical formation of the global care market. The answers for why migrant domestic care workers have become the favorite choice of surrogate caregiver for families lie in the Taiwanese migrant labour policy. Therefore, migrant labour policy is examined to show how migrant domestic care workers are systematically excluded from the protection of labour laws against the risks of abuse and mistreatments. In short, the traditional Confucian family ethic gives Taiwanese women the primary role as caregivers in the family, while migrant labour policy renders migrant female labour available for Taiwanese women to fulfill their moral obligation as daughters-in-law. These forces set the context for the power relations within the households.

In the second part of the chapter, we look at four cases of Taiwanese households with Filipina workers to explore the conflicts, tension, and struggles between daughters-in-law and migrant care workers and to demonstrate how gender, class, and race intersect in the daily lives of Taiwanese households that hire migrant care workers. The war between women for their care work in the household has been the key reproductive mechanism by which women are subjugated into the role of caregiver. The old war between daughter-in-law and mother-in-law in Chinese family discourse has its modern version in the relation of daughter-in-law and migrant care worker. What remains unchanged is that wars over domestic work are always wars among women.

## The Daughter-in-Law in the Traditional Three-Generational Family Discourse

In the Chinese family tradition, caring for frail people has long been defined as a family responsibility, and therefore a woman's responsibility (Hu 1995). However, since this hegemonic family ideology has been challenged since the political democratisation process, which began in the late 1980s, the resulting changes in ideology have implications for policy formation and enforcement. The traditional Confucian ideas of family ethics enable the Taiwanese government to play a minimal role in the provision of long-term care, by defining elder care as a private responsibility. The government provides institutional care only to a strictly defined population, namely those elders who are poor and without family. Any attempt to expand the role of government in long-term care is interpreted as a threat to the traditional family value system. It was not surprising, then, that responding to a request from the opposition party for a public care system for the elderly in the early 1990s, former Premier Ho replied that "The three-generation-family is the ideal type of family in Taiwan and the promotion of this ideal type of family should be the future of Chinese elder care" (*United Daily News*, 14 September 1991).

The ideal Chinese family system has long been recognised as a perfect example of patrilineal patriarchy (Hamilton 1990; Gates 1987). Only males were heirs; female children were seen as only a temporary part of the family, and thus were trained in household skills so they could be married into a friendly, rich, and powerful household (Copper 1990). A man and his sons and grandsons, forming a property-owning corporation, ideally lived together in a continuously expanding household that might encompass the proverbial 'five generations under one roof.' This image of the multi-gener-ational family has been the symbol of a secure old age for Chinese elderly people because the large number of young men and their potential wives represents the amount of caring labour available. In the patrilineal version of kinship relations, women take a distinctly and overtly inferior place. Because a daughter is considered to be less valuable than a son, almost not a member of the family, her only legitimate destiny is to marry and become a mother in some other family.[2] A married woman is expected to act as a humble, servant-like daughter to her parents-in-law and to obey her moth-er-in-law in everything. Warm and affectionate relations between wife and husband are to be concealed, if they develop, for fear of the mother-in-law's jealous disapproval, in that the security of her old age depends on her son.

With the birth of a son, the daughter-in-law will strengthen her status in her husband's family; the status of a daughter-in-law depends upon the number of sons she gives birth to. With the arrival of a daughter-in-law, a woman achieves a position of authority as mother-in-law and her life improves with the onset of old age (Gallin 1994; Gates 1987). This trans-formation of daughter-in-law into mother-in-law had been normalised as a pattern of living for most Chinese women, a consistent mutually abusive relationship between old and young female generations. A vicious cycle of women's oppression is constructed to extract women's caring labour into the family, with women both the oppressor and the oppressed (Hu 1995). The patriarchal family structure positions different cohorts of women into competition for men's affection and, in that competition, the family is pro-vided with the necessary caring labour.

Taiwanese married women are under constant surveillance as wives and daughters-in-law, according to their care work in the family. Those who fail to obey the norm of submissive daughter-in-law and to provide care to family members are labelled as 'un-dutiful daughter-in-law.' The well-established images of obedient daughter-in-law and harsh mother-in-law are deeply rooted in the fables and slang of Taiwanese society and have become the norm for examining women's practices of care within the family. When an elderly person is in need of care, "where is his/her family?" is the question raised and, in fact, it is the daughter-in-law who is scrutinised and examined.

In practice today, as the rapid economic development in the past four decades has increased female labour participation to more than 50 per-cent, it is increasingly more difficult for Taiwanese women to stay at home to carry out all the care tasks, compared to the traditional agricultural economy; nevertheless it remains women's responsibility to manage care work within the family. Finding substitute care becomes the strategy for the daughters-in-law who cannot or will not care for the family by themselves. Therefore, the need for substitutes has become a growing market, as Taiwanese women have been incorporated into the labour market since the 1960s, when Taiwan's economy started the process of industrialisation.

## THE GLOBALISATION OF THE CARE MARKET

With increasing rates of female employment and aging populations and the gendered cultural expectation of family care, providing care has become difficult in most societies (Taylor-Gooby 2004). The lack of public intervention has turned the rising needs for elder care into a profitable market with varying levels of care and cost.

Although the Taiwanese government has been expanding the public subsidised home care for elderly people since the 1980s, its target population has mainly been low-income elderly persons. Public subsidised home care has been available to all since 2004, but a 40 percent co-payment requirement has made home care less attractive than the employment of migrant domestic care workers. Compared with the needs for elder care, the supply of public subsidised home care and nursing homes is insignificant. The importation of migrant domestic care workers, i.e., the cheapest care, since 1992, has made migrant workers the primary providers of home care. The 2000 Population and Housing Census (Directorate-General of Budget, Accounting and Statistics 2000) shows that there were 182,351 elderly persons in need of care and only 8 percent of them were institutionalised. Among those living in the community, 78 percent of them lived with their families. At the same time, there were 74,793 migrant care workers reported to be living in Taiwan in 1999. These care workers were estimated to provide care for approximately 40 percent of the elderly persons in need of long-term care in Taiwan (Lo, Yu, and Wu 2007). The number of migrant care workers working at home to care for frail adults reached 183,573 in 2010, a figure that is almost 2.45 times the figure in 1999 (see Table 7.1). A recent study from the supply side shows an even more significant proportion of migrant care workers. Chen and Wu (2004) reported that the capacity of institutional care was 56,038 and that of public subsidised home care was 28,138, with a total capacity of 84,176. However, the total number of migrant workers was 135,659 in 2004, or about two thirds of the capacity provided by the long-term care system in Taiwan.

Migrant labour policy has become the most decisive force in shaping the organisation of the long-term care system in Taiwan. The cultural expectation 'pulls' families to keep the elderly member at home. Yet, the lack of public long-term care policy 'pushes' families to turn to the market where

*Table 7.1*  Number of Migrant Workers in Taiwan (1992 to 2010)

| | Total migrant workers | Care Workers | | | |
|---|---|---|---|---|---|
| | | Total | Care workers (in nursing home) | Domestic care workers (at home) | Home helpers |
| 1992 | 15,924 | 669 | | 306 | 363 |
| 1995 | 189,051 | 17,407 | | 8,902 | 8,505 |
| 1998 | 270,620 | 53,368 | | 41,844 | 11,524 |
| 2001 | 304,605 | 112,934 | 2,653 | 101,127 | 9,154 |
| 2004 | 314,034 | 131,067 | 5,066 | 123,157 | 2,844 |
| 2007 | 357,937 | 162,228 | 7,635 | 152,067 | 2,526 |
| 2010 (up to August) | 372,146 | 183,573 | 9,280 | 172,002 | 2,291 |

*Source:* Commission of Labour Affairs (2010)

the migrant worker is the cheapest and most available type of care.[3] The sheer number of applications far exceeds the current capacity of the long-term care system. The needs for elderly care therefore take the different path of privatisation, not through the family, based on Confucian teaching, but through the market, via a transnational exchange of caring labours, which Hochschild (2000) called 'global care chains.'

## MIGRANT CARE WORKER POLICIES THAT PRODUCE DOCILE CARING LABOUR

Facing competition from China, Taiwanese employers put pressure on the government to address the lack of labour force and lobbied for importation of migrant workers to enhance 'national competitiveness' in the early 1990s. Although Liu (2000) argues that the so-called lack of 'labour' is in fact lack of 'cheap and exploitable' labour, the Taiwanese government decided to import migrant workers in 1992 for the sake of "compensating for a shortage of local labour" (59). The migrant worker policy adopted the 'guest worker' principle that they will not be granted permanent resident status, in order to prevent permanent settlement. The government introduced a system of quota control and contract employment to regulate the number and the length of stay of migrant workers. These regulatory measures deprive migrant workers of their basic rights as workers.

As guest workers, migrant workers face multiple constraints which leave them in a very inferior position to bargain with their employers. Migrant workers are not free labourers in the market, as they cannot quit their jobs. As migrant workers cannot change employers and the renewal of their contract depends on their employer's consent, migrant workers find it difficult to say no to their employers. In addition, migrant workers cannot join unions, they cannot use collective bargaining power with employers, nor do they have a right to strike. Migrant workers residence is also time-limited because they cannot stay longer than nine years. Worst of all, their working conditions are not covered by the Labour Standard Law, which guarantees workers' basic rights. Therefore, the working hours and job description are left for migrant domestic workers to negotiate with their employers individually. In such an unequal power relationship, it is very difficult for migrant workers to refuse employers' requests, both reasonable and unreasonable.

The scope of importation is limited to certain industries and occupations. Soon after the importation of manufacturing workers began, the government immediately added the second type of migrant worker, the 'migrant care worker.' This migrant care worker policy is presented by the government as a cost-saving solution to the growing demands for paid childcare and eldercare among the growing number of nuclear households and the aging population. Therefore, the policy is considered a type of 'welfare.' Ironically, this welfare is not provided by the state, but by the market; what the government does is simply grant the families the right to access the market.

Each migrant care worker can stay in Taiwan no longer than nine years, with an initial permit lasting for three years, and a maximum of two extensions if the employer is willing to apply. Employers have to pay the 'Stable Employment Fee' of NT$2,000 (US$67) per month to the government in order to compensate for the possible loss of employment opportunities for local Taiwanese workers. The total cost is thus about NT$20,000 (US$595) per month. Despite the qualification of employers being subject to strict regulations, the number of Taiwanese families employing migrant domestic care workers has rapidly increased within the past seventeen years (see Table 7.1). Currently over 180,000 migrant workers, coming from Indonesia, the Philippines, and Vietnam, are legally employed as domestic workers in Taiwan (Labour Affairs Commission 2010).

There are two types of migrant care workers. The government granted work permits in 1992 to 'domestic care workers' who were employed to provide personal care for the severely ill or disabled. This has become the major type of migrant care worker (over 90 percent). In the same year, the government allowed a small quota for the employment of 'home helpers,' the so-called nanny or maid, to households with children under the age of twelve or elderly members above the age of seventy. There is a distinction between domestic care worker and home helper; the former provides personal care to the disabled or patients while the latter helps with household chores and childcare. However, such distinctions are usually blurred in practice. Many households apply for domestic care workers, but then assign them household chores or childcare, or vice versa. It does not matter how a migrant worker comes into the household. Once they are in the house, they care for all members of the family.

The rise of the care market indicates a different form of privatisation of care work. Since caring for family members is defined as a family responsibility, managing migrant workers is also considered part of this family responsibility. To minimise management costs for the state, and to prohibit migrant workers from permanent settlement, the government requires employers to oversee migrant workers. If the migrant worker should run away, the employer is obliged to inform the police and locate the worker, and the employer is penalised, losing the right to apply for another migrant care worker until the previous worker is caught.[4] Government policy has thus created fear among the employers about their migrants potentially running away, and has divided Taiwanese women and migrant care workers into supervisors and subordinates (Lin 2009).

This tension between employers and migrant workers provides an opportunity for the broker to construct migrant care workers based on their ethnicity. Lan (2000) reported that Taiwanese brokers tend to construct racially stereotyped images of migrant domestic workers to manipulate employers' perceptions of the migrant workers in order to have a docile worker with minimum risk of running away. For instance, Filipina workers are portrayed as troublesome but capable of speaking English, which is good for teaching children; workers from Vietnam are seen as obedient, culturally similar, and therefore adaptable to the local lifestyle; Indonesian workers are construed as docile but lacking in good hygiene habits due to their background as peasants from rural areas. Yet, in fact, Vietnamese workers have the highest rate of running away in Taiwan. What is made invisible behind this racial construction of migrant care workers is the different transnational organisation of the migrant worker market which offers various commission rates to the local brokers. Such racialised portrayal of migrant care workers allows the broker to manipulate the hiring behaviours of employers. What is missing from the scene is that these stereotyped images of migrant care workers are, in fact, tightly linked with the calculation of profitability among migrant workers, which is shaped by the political economy of the international migrant worker brokerage trade.

## POWER RELATIONS WITHIN THE HOUSEHOLD: ARE WE SISTERS STRUGGLING AGAINST EACH OTHER?

We will look at four cases of Filipina domestic workers working for Taiwanese households to explore the power relations between wives/daughters-in-law and domestic workers in the household. The following analysis is based on interviews conducted by the second author with members of the four households: the Lees, the Changs, the Wangs, and the Hos (all pseudonyms) (see Table 7.2), and their domestic workers (see Table 7.3). These Filipina domestic workers were recruited as home helpers, that is, nannies for children, but in reality they cared for all members within the household, or worked as maids for the family.

*Table 7.2* Data of Interviewed Households

| Wife – Maid | Mrs. Lee – Regina | Mrs. Chang – Rosemarie | Mrs. Wang – Grace | Mrs. Ho – Nancy |
|---|---|---|---|---|
| Employment status of the wife | housewife | housewife | work full-time | work full-time |
| Management style | emotional control | emotional control | business-like relationships | business-like relationships |
| Family type | nuclear family | nuclear family | live with parents-in-law | nuclear family |

*Table 7.3* Data of Interviewed Migrant Workers

| Name | Age | Marital status, children | Education | Previous job | First job abroad | Residence in Taiwan |
|---|---|---|---|---|---|---|
| Regina | 41 | Married, 2 | University | Ran her business | Yes | 10 months |
| Rosemarie | 30s | Married, 3 | Junior and vocational course | Owner of beauty salon | Yes | 1 year, 7 months |
| Grace | 31 | Married, 4 | University (incomplete) | Housekeeper | Yes | 2 years |
| Nancy | 30s | Married, 4 | University (incomplete) | Office staff, domestic worker in Hong Kong | No | 10 months |

## THE FEELING OF GUILT AMONG DAUGHTERS-IN-LAW

When a Filipina domestic worker was hired, the care work would be re-arranged among the women in the household. Both Mrs. Lee and Mrs. Chang were full-time housewives responsible for managing the domestic labour and childcare before employing a Filipina domestic worker. Their husbands were successful in business and spent little time at home. Mrs. Wang and Mrs. Ho worked full-time. Mrs. Wang had her mother-in-law to care for her child, while finding a nanny became Mrs. Ho's task. The gender division of labour followed the rigid man-as-breadwinner pattern. After each of these women employed a domestic worker, the domestic work gradually becomes the maids' work. The employers became house-managers, with all the heavy and routine jobs done by the domestic workers.

However, the domestic workers do not exempt daughters-in-law from the duty of domestic labour. No matter how privileged and wealthy she appears, a daughter-in-law or a wife in a Chinese family is expected to keep house and to care for the family members with love. Taiwanese women not only bear these expectations but also internalise these ideas of what a 'good woman' should do. Therefore, when they do not perform housework and caring roles at home by themselves, they feel guilty. Both Mrs. Lee and Mrs. Chang thought that they were still doing the housework because Mrs. Lee now could 'make more cookies' and Mrs. Chang had more time 'playing with children and being in a good mood.' This shows their anxiety in employing maids to perform the work that they are 'supposed' to do. Likewise, Mrs. Wang felt guilty if she did not help the mother-in-law do the domestic work and Mrs. Ho also felt guilty about her children if she could not take care of them because of her work. Hidden behind these women's guilt are the social expectations of women carrying out housework and child/elderly care.

Domestic labour is considered women's work, and is always shifting from women to women: from mother-in-law to daughter-in-law, and from wife to maid. The war between daughter-in-law and migrant worker is a re-activation of the old war between mother-in-law and daughter-in-law. The script is the same. In this sense, all women share the same structural position to do domestic labour. Women in power are always trying to download the care work to the 'other' women. It was the daughter-in-law, who was the woman from the 'other' family, in the three-generation family discourse; but now it is the migrant worker, who is the woman from the 'other' country, in the global chain of care. Yet, the existence of a Filipina maid does not free Taiwanese women from domestic labour. The gendered construction of domestic labour has not yet changed. The daughter-in-law is still expected to supervise the maid's work and to fill in when the maid is off.

## IF LOVE/SEX + LABOUR = WIFE, WHAT'S THE DIFFERENCE BETWEEN US?

In addition to the physical labour, a wife performs emotional labour in the family. Emotional labour is regarded as the most special characteristic of a wife. A wife is different from a maid because she does domestic labour with love. If the live-in domestic worker provides emotional labour, would the maid replace the daughter-in-law?

The Filipina domestic worker provides emotional labour, especially when she is responsible for caring for children or the elderly. The maid usually develops strong ties with her charges. Therefore, any interaction implying intimacy between the male employer and the Filipina domestic worker becomes threatening to the wife who fears losing her position as a wife if the domestic worker becomes a competitor. Any ambivalent emotional and physical crossing must be prevented. Therefore, brokers always give advice to the maid to keep away from their male employers: "The agencies told me to have good relationship with daughter-in-law. If she likes you, you can stay long. And, not be close to the master. It's true" (Regina). The Filipina maids were also well aware of the tension between them and their female employers:

> "The agency told us that most important was when dealing with the wives, not to provoke jealousy in respect to the husband. Many cases abroad, like in Singapore or Middle East, mostly the madam of the domestic helper is jealous with [of] them, because they [the maid] are very close to the men, their boss. So . . . It's not good to be close to the men, it's better to be close to the wives, so that you can stay longer" (Nancy).

The wives had various levels of anxiety about the perceived relationships between the maids and the husbands. Mrs. Wang did not worry since her parents-in-law were always present at home. Her confidence was built on her perception of the otherness of the maid. She thought that the Filipina maid was so different from the Taiwanese that there was little chance for her husband to fall for the maid. Mrs. Lee and Mrs. Chang worried less because their husbands had few chances to be in contact with the domestic workers. Mrs. Ho did worry about the possibility but she felt powerless because she spent much of her time working outside the home. The domestic worker, who sensed the underlying tension between them, kept her distance from the husband. This pattern shows how the maid and daughter-in-law relationship is reproducing the competing relationship between the two groups of women.

The same pattern of competition between women also occurs in the relationship between the mother-in-law and the daughter-in-law in the Chinese family. As the son is in charge of all resources, affectionate relations between wife and husband are to be concealed, for fear of the mother-in-law's jealous disapproval. Similarly, as the male is the main breadwinner, his affections will determine a woman's position within the family. It is possible that the maid could win his affection and further replace the wife. The old pattern of mothers-in-law abusing their daughters-in-law is reproduced in the relation between daughter-in-law and migrant worker. A consistent, mutually abusive relationship between old and young female generations is now expanded into women of two nations as well as two classes. A vicious cycle of women's oppression is reproduced to extract women's caring labour into the family, with women both the oppressor and the oppressed. The patriarchal family structure ensures that the man secures the financial safety and thus positions different nations of women into competition for the man's affection. In that competition among women, the family is provided with the necessary caring labour.

## "WE ARE A FAMILY, AREN'T WE?"

As Fung (1952) pointed out, the traditional Chinese family system was one of the most complex and well organised in the world. The Chinese have developed a complicated system of addressing each other to reflect the hierarchy of authority within the family, based on gender and age. The superior persons can call the inferior ones by their first name, while the superior ones must be addressed by their titles. Proper practices of address are considered part of the basic manners for a Chinese person (Jacobs 1990). As an outsider within the family, the maid needs a name to be present within the family. How the maid is addressed reflects her position within the family and how her behaviours will be interpreted. In our interviews, all the daughters-in-law claimed that the Filipina maid was a member of the family. To claim that the maid is a member of the family made her role as a worker invisible. What was not revealed was how the maids were ranked the lowest within the family hierarchy, as reflected in the ways they were addressed.

The maids are told by brokers to call their female employer 'Mom,' male employer 'Sir,' mother-in-law of the female employer 'Amah' (grandmother), and father-in-law 'Agong' (grandfather), as a gesture of respect towards the adults in the family. However, these practices of address construct the maid as the lowest rank in the family, as the child. Accordingly, all the family members, adults or children alike, call her by her first name, thus positioning the maid at the lowest level of the family hierarchy, the same as the position of a child. 'Mom' seems to imply an intimate relation with her female employer, but also implies unconditional subordination to the teachings of her female employer. The addresses used in the household already suggest that she is a degraded and secondary family member. The Filipina maid is usually of an age similar to her female employer, but the latter does not regard her as 'my sister'; rather, she requires the maid to call her 'Mom.' This hierarchical practice implies the class differences between them and the fact that the maid should subordinate herself to the daughter-in-law as a daughter is subordinate to her mother.

According to the Chinese customs of address, a female adult in their twenties or thirties, like the maids are, should be called 'aunt.' Therefore, when the children call her by her name it is an act of transgression of the kinship hierarchy in which the maid is degraded. However, from the view point of Filipino culture, calling one by name is an act of closeness and friendship, so this is acceptable to the Filipina maids. Being called by their first names does not insult their dignity as adults; however, for a Taiwanese child, calling the maid by her name implies transgression of age hierarchy and shows disrespect to her role in the family.

The lack of status within the family is apparent for Nancy. When her contract was about to expire, she was not informed until one week before the date of expiration. She complained, saying, "My mom says she loves me. She says I am a member of the family. But they are going to send me home without informing me." This is part of the power that the daughter-in-law is given by the state apparatus, in that only the employer can apply for extension of the work permit. The power relations between the daughter-in-law and the maid are not merely a result of discursive formation, but are supported by policies that deprive Filipina workers of their rights to quit a job, bargain for wages, form a union, or go on strike. In addition, all migrant workers have had to take on heavy debt to come and work abroad, which makes them unable to say no to their employers.

## DEGRADED AS A FILIPINA MAID

As a guest worker, job security for migrant care workers depends on the will of their employers, which is the source of unequal power relations with the daughter-in-law. A Filipina domestic worker carries out degrading domestic labour in the household, under unequal power relations as a member of the lowest class, and she is also degraded for her race as a Filipina. In the Foreign Domestic Helper Habit Guide, which is provided by the broker for the employer, the image of a Filipina domestic worker is connected with dirt, as they are seen as a source of disease. It starts with their sanitary habits. They are told to brush teeth, wash their hands with soap, take a shower every day, and trim fingernails and toenails, etc. This reflects the Taiwanese imagination that non-white foreigners come from under-developed areas and, therefore, the first thing they need to learn is to keep clean. The second part of the guidance is about the living etiquette at home and at public. At home, they are told to obey employers' requests and to try to please the visitors. In public, they are told to wear neat clothes, not to litter, keep out of mischief, not to make noise in public places, obey traffic regulations, and so on. These instructions are quite common in children's school textbooks. The efforts to 'educate' Filipina maids with such teachings reveal the fact that the Taiwanese people regard Filipino workers as 'uncivilised' and 'uneducated' foreigners. This perception is far removed from the reality, namely that Filipina domestic workers are well-educated workers from a 'westernised/civilised' country.

Many domestic workers feel that they are looked down upon and degraded. Regina had degrading experiences as a Filipina domestic helper. She ate with her employers at home, but when the family went out to eat, she had to stand and serve them. Her employer degraded her by showing her off to his friends. In front of his friends, the employer asked her to clean after a dog, which was not her responsibility. Regina was very embarrassed and then her employer and friends laughed at her. She was degraded through the metaphor of a dog and dirt by being asked to make the dirt unseen (to clean the shit). These degrading situations are unlikely to happen to Taiwanese maids.

## MANAGING THE OTHER WOMEN AT HOME AS BUSINESS

Within the four households, Mrs. Ho and Mrs. Wang worked full-time and spent a great deal of time at work, while Mrs. Lee and Mrs. Chang were housewives with strong networks and very rich social lives. Looking at their relationships with the domestic workers, and borrowing Romero's (1992) concepts, we categorise the former two as having 'business-like' relationships and the latter two as having a pattern of 'emotional control.' The daughters-in-law had different managing styles towards the maids.

In the business-like style, the daughters-in-law had less time at home to supervise, so there was little communication between the employee and the employer. This relationship may be good for a live-out domestic worker but it was problematic in the context of the live-in domestic worker. The lack of trust and communication between them meant that the relationship could be difficult to sustain, due to suspicions or conflicts.

Mrs. Wang maintained a business-like relationship with her domestic worker, Grace. They rarely communicated with each other and Mrs. Wang did not trust Grace. When the family members suspected Grace of stealing something, Mrs. Wang did not respond with emotion; instead she dealt with this rationally. Since nothing important was lost, she decided it was not important and ignored the complaints. She said, "I don't know whether she stole something or not. But, I have to believe that she did not. I tell myself that if I did not find something lost, that thing must be not important for me. Otherwise, I will have to stay at home looking after her all the time."

The business-like relationship is also reflected in the employer's decision on workers' days of leave. Mrs. Wang felt that Grace's workload was not heavy so she gave Grace only one day off a month. Grace had no say in this. When Grace asked for one more day off, Mrs. Wang was angry and prohibited her from receiving any phone calls. The daughter-in-law exercised her power over the maid to display her authority and reinforce the class differences. Mrs. Wang later decided not to extend Grace's contract. She regrets that she failed to maintain strict criteria from the beginning to make Grace a good worker. If Mrs. Wang could start again, she would like to stick to a clear work schedule and defined tasks for her maid. That is in line with her business-like management style.

The Hos stayed at home less than twelve hours a day, and they also had a business-like relationship with Nancy. Nancy had a heavy workload but she was not supervised and had some freedom when the employer worked outside the home. The communication between the worker and the employer was limited. Living under the same roof but having limited conversation made Nancy feel that she was different and was not trusted by her employers. However, one benefit for the maid in a business-like relationship is that the maid can maintain her privacy away from the employer's intrusion.

## EMOTIONAL WORK BY THE DAUGHTER-IN-LAW

In contrast to the distant and suspicious business-like relationship, Mrs. Lee and Mrs. Chang had a much more emotional involvement with their domestic workers. Both of them were housewives so they were able to spend a lot of time with their children and their domestic workers. Harmony is the guiding principle for the Chinese in dealing with interpersonal relations. Deeply influenced by the cultural expectation of being a good woman, they said that domestic work was their responsibility and they just employed maids to 'share' it. A good woman is expected to manage interpersonal relationships within the household harmoniously. Mrs. Lee and Mrs. Chang paid a lot of attention to their maids and maintained a good relationship with them. The cultural expectation of managing interpersonal relations in harmony provides a counter-force to balance the institutional tendency to abuse migrant care worker and makes Mrs. Lee and Mrs. Chang 'good employers.' They considered the issue of "how to manage and have good relationship with the maid" as important as having good relationships with their husband and children. Both maids mentioned that they were treated as a member of the family and had very good relationships with their mistresses. Mrs. Lee and Mrs. Chang showed their affections to their maids because an equal and respectful relationship freed them from the feeling that they were oppressing another woman. Their relationship was based on the reciprocal exchange of labour and affection. These cases reveal that the workload and emotional support are two different things and not necessarily related. Even though the employer may be emotionally attached to the domestic worker, the workload may not necessarily be reduced.

Nevertheless, their management style was a dynamic process and covered a range between business-like and emotional control, rather than being a fixed dichotomy for the Taiwanese daughter-in-law. Mrs. Lee is a good example. Mrs. Lee did not have a maid until she employed a Filipina maid and later employed four such maids. She explained how she learned to adjust to the relationship with a maid. At first, she had very loose expectations of the first maid, and the only clear one was for the maid to take care of the youngest daughter when Mrs. Lee was busy. Mrs. Lee tried to show respect to her Filipina maids so she used 'Miss Finipina' to refer to the Filipina workers, while the common usage in Taiwan is 'Filipina maid.' She also took care of her maid, taking a personal interest in her,

her background, her family, her friends, etc. When she was out, she would bring home a McDonald's hamburger for the maid. She said that she was very nervous about having a maid. However, that was quite an emotional burden for both sides. Having employed four different maids, she learned not to treat the maid as her child in need of protection, and moved instead towards the pole of a business-like style. She gave the maid certain jobs, was concerned only about her work performance, and did not need to know about all the relatives and life concerns of the maid in order to prove that they were a family.

## PEER SUPPORT AND GOING HOME

Being unprivileged and doing degrading work as foreign maids in Taiwan, Filipina domestic workers suffer from homesickness, stress, depression, and loneliness. But the comforts of meeting other Filipinos, their belief in God and attending Sunday mass, the support from family in the Philippines, and sometimes the affection for their charges give them strength to continue their work. The Filipino support network plays a very important role in their working lives in Taiwan and was mentioned over and over in the interviews.

> Of course people cry. Not only me, also my daughter, also my husband. Sad and very lonely. But, even [when] I feel so lonely, I went to church. I talked to the priest, I talked [about] my problem. Of course, it's a problem, right? Yeah, and the Father told me, 'oh, you just pray. You ask our Lord.' After [that], I pray. No, no more problems. In the [Taipei] Train Station, sometimes we talk about the lives, and, after that, the funny stories. We laugh, laugh, all day long. Sometimes I went to the park to take pictures and send [to] my husband, send [to] my daughter, just like that. (Rosemarie)

Meeting with peers creates a public space that belongs to Filipina maids to share their problems and stories. "Because we miss our homeland in the Philippines, so every Saturday I am very happy. Tomorrow is Sunday, I am going out and I feel relax. If I meet Filipino, we [are] just like in the Philippines. That's why we like to meet each other" (Regina). The collective gathering of migrant workers has transformed certain public areas, such as the Taipei Train Station, into a Filipino space during Sundays, so much so that even Taiwanese feel they are strangers in that space (Wang, forthcoming).

When Filipina domestic workers feel really unhappy, they make use of the final tactic they have left, returning home, to resist the oppressive system. Going home implies that there is still an alternative in their lives. Although few workers do go home, the knowledge that they could has provided them with the strength to prove that they still have some dignity as a

Filipina worker in Taiwan. However, money is the major issue that blocks their return home. Although Taiwan offers higher wages for migrant workers than most Asian countries[6] (NT$15,840 (US$528) per month), migrant workers often must go deeply into debt to pay the broker's fees and need to pay that back before they can start making any money. The 'payment' in Grace's account was her major concern in the decision to go home. "Even she [the daughter-in-law] said that 'don't go home until you finish your work,' but I miss home. It's payment, anyway. I have already [earned] half of my payment. The other half, if they want me to go home, it's OK for me. I can see my family" (Grace).

In Regina's case, her family encouraged her to go home and was willing to reimburse her financial loss. But she was struggling to stay and wished to find a good employer, so she could stay. "My father, they gave me financial aid already. I am about going home, but still not yet finish . . . They said, 'you'd better come home and you will be happier.' Because my children miss me, but, if only I found a good employer, I would not thinking of going home. That time I signed the contract, it was my desire to work for two years" (Regina). In her account, whether she would be able to earn money during her time in Taiwan depends on her luck to have a good employer, somewhat akin to the lottery. The words "if only I" fully demonstrate the lack of control and power on the side of migrant workers within the family as well as within the global system of care.

## CONCLUSION

The cultural ideas of family ethics and the migrant care worker policy result in the same political effects of re-producing women into docile caring labour. In the family discourse, a married woman is expected to act as a humble, servant-like daughter to her parents-in-law and to obey her mother-in-law in everything. As guest workers, migrant workers face multiple constraints which leave them in a very inferior position from which to bargain with their employers. Such an unequal power relationship renders the migrant workers unable to refuse employers' requests. When the daughter-in-law encounters the migrant care worker, a new hierarchy among women is formed based on race and class. Migrant care workers take the position of daughter-in-law who provides care, while daughters-in-law move into a managerial position similar to that of mother-in-law. A consistent, mutually abusive relationship between old and young female generations has now expanded to include women from other countries. Multiple vicious cycles of women's oppression are constructed to extract women's caring labour into the family, with women both the oppressor and the oppressed. However, we also find that the cultural expectation of a good woman to maintain all interpersonal relationships in harmony can become a counter-force to transform the female employer into a good employer.

In general, the employers are not mean and keen on exploitation. However, both parties are locked into a vicious cycle created by policies that portray migrant workers as 'the other,' which legitimises the deprivation of their basic rights. This is similar to the construction of the image of the un-dutiful daughter-in-law, whereby women are designated to provide care work, therefore reinforcing gender inequality. Both forces transform structural oppression into interpersonal conflicts. The concept of the 'un-dutiful daughter-in-law' divides women according to age by their role as mother-in-law and daughter-in-law, with the former competing against the latter for the son's affection. The construction of the migrant worker as 'maid' divides women according to race and class based on their role as employer and domestic worker, with the former supervising the latter in constant fear that the worker will replace her position as the wife. Such patterns have gone on for too long without recognition.

## NOTES

1. The term 'migrant care worker' is used in the general sense to refer to those migrant workers who provide care to patients, elderly or disabled persons, or children in the home setting or in institutions. It will be used interchangeably with terms such as domestic worker, maid, and nanny.
2. This patrilineal determination of women's roles is reflected in the division of caring tasks for elderly family members between daughters and daughters-in-law. When an elderly family member is in need of care, unmarried daughters can choose not to share the work while daughters-in-law have no option but to take on the role of caregivers. The logic is that daughters are supposed to care for elderly members of their husbands' families. In other words, daughters are viewed by Chinese parents as daughters-in-law of other families.
3. The Council of Labour Affairs (CLA) tried to integrate the long-term care system into the needs assessment process in 2005 as a way to regulate the rapid increase in migrant workers. However, the developmental nature of the welfare state and the reluctance to invest in the elderly and the disabled have resulted in an under-developed public care system that lacks effective management of needs assessment.
4. The whole regulation has been abolished since 2008, but this regulation has had a major impact on the relationship between employers and migrant workers, and provides important context for the cases discussed below.
5. Names that appear are all changed to protect the interviewees.
6. Hong Kong is said to offer the highest wage to migrant care worker. The official minimum wage for foreign maids in Hong Kong was $460 (HK$3,580) in 2011.

## BIBLIOGRAPHY

Chen, Hui-Zi & Wu, Xiao-Qi (2005). Manpower supply and demand in long-term care analysis and estimation. Report for the Long Term Care Planning Committee, Council of Economic Development, Executive Yuan, Taiwan. (in Chinese).
Commission of Labour Affairs (2010) 'Statistics of Migrant Worker.' http://statdb.cla.gov.tw/statis/webproxy.aspx?sys=100&funid=alienjsp. Retrieved on

6 January 2010. http://www.evta.gov.tw/files/57/724052.csv. Retrieved on 20 September 2010.

Copper, J. F. (1990) *Taiwan: Nation-State or Province?* Boulder, San Francisco, London: Westview Press, Inc.

Daly, M., and J. Lewis (2000) 'The Concept of Social Care and the Analysis of Contemporary Welfare States.' *British Journal of Sociology*, 51(2): 281.

Directorate-General of Budget, Accounting and Statistics (2000) '2000 Population and Housing Census.' Executive Yuan, R.O.C. http://eng.stat.gov.tw/public/Data/511114261371.rtf. Retrieved on 26 January 2010.

Fung, Y. L. (1952). *A history of Chinese philosophy*. Princeton: Princeton University Press.

Gallin, R. S. (1994) 'The Intersection of Class and Age: Mother-in-law/Daughter-in-law Relations in Rural Taiwan.' *Journal of Cross-Cultural Gerontology*, 9: 127–40.

Gates, H. (1987). 'Chinese Working-class Lives: Getting By in Taiwan'. Ithaca, London: Cornell University Press.

Hamilton, G. G. (1990). 'Patriarchy, Patrimonialism, and Filial Piety: A Comparison of China and Western Europe'. *British Journal of Sociology*, 41(1), 77–104.

Hochschild, A. R. (2000) 'Global Care Chains and Emotional Surplus Value.' In *On The Edge: Living with Global Capitalism*, edited by W. Hutton and A. Giddens, 130–46. London: Jonathan Cape.

Holliday, I. (2000) 'Productivist Welfare Capitalism: Social Policy in East Asia.' *Political Studies*, 48(4): 706.

Hu, Y. H. (1995) *Three-Generation-Family: Myths and Traps*. Taipei: Chui-Liu Publishing, Inc.

Jacobs, J. (1990) 'Names, Naming, and Name Calling in Practice with Families.' *Journal of Contemporary Human Services*, 71(7): 415–21.

Jones, C. (1993) 'The Pacific Challenge-Confucian Welfare States.' In *New Perspectives on the Welfare State in Europe*, edited by C. Jones, 198–217. London: Routledge.

Ku, Y. W. (1995). The development of state welfare in the Asian NICs with special reference to Taiwan. *Social Policy & Administration*, 29(4), 345–364.

Kwon, H.-J. (2005) 'Transforming the Developmental Welfare State in East Asia.' *Development & Change*, 36(3): 477–97.

Lan, Pei-Chia (2000). *Global Divisions, Local Identities: Filipina Migrant Domestic Workers and Taiwanese Employers*. Ph.D. Dissertation, Department of Sociology, Northwestern University, Evanston, IL.

Lee, Y.-J., and Y.-W. Ku (2007) 'East Asian Welfare Regimes: Testing the Hypothesis of the Developmental Welfare State.' *Social Policy & Administration*, 41(2):197–212.

Lin, C.-J. (2009) 'The State Policy that Divided Women: Rethinking Feminist Critiques to "The Foreign Maid Policy" in Taiwan.' In *Taishe Reader in Immigration*, edited by H.-C. Hsia, 425–72. Taipei: Taishe.

Liu, M.-C. (2000) 'A Critique from Marxist Political Economy on the Cheap Foreign Labour Discourse.' *Taiwan: A Radical Quarterly in Social Studies*, 38: 59–90.

Lo, Joan C., Suchuan Yu and Su-Feng Wu (2007) "An Exploratory Investigation on the Care Takers Cared by Foreign Workers," in Joan C. Lo (ed. *The Study of Foreign Workers in Taiwan*, p. 129–154 Taipei Institute of Economics, Academia Sinica. (in Chinese)

Romero, M. (1992) *Maid in the U.S.A.* New York: Routledge.

Taylor-Gooby, P. & J. Kananen (2004). 'New Social Risks in Post-Industrial Society', *International Social Security Review*, 57(3), 45–64.

Wang, C.-H. (Forthcoming) 'Do We Have a Multi-cultural City? The Southeast Asian Ethnic Territorialization in Taipei Metropolitan Area.' *Taiwan: A Radical Quarterly in Social Studies*.

Wang, H.-Z. (2009) 'In Whose Interests? Transnational Labour Migration System between Vietnam and Taiwan.' In Tais*he Reader in Im/migration,* edited by H.-C. Hsia, 201–27. Taipei: Taishe.

Williams, F. (2003) 'Rethinking Care in Social Policy.' Paper given at the Annual Conference of the Finnish Social Policy Association, University of Joensuu, Finland, 24 October 2003.

Wong, W. (1981) 'The Impacts of Chinese Family Concepts to Political Democratization.' Master's thesis, Graduate School of Sun Yat-Senism, National Taiwan University.

# Part IV

# Transnational Social Support and Biography

# 8 Migration Biographies and Transnational Social Support
## Transnational Family Care and the Search for 'Homelandmen'

*Désirée Bender, Tina Hollstein, Lena Huber, and Cornelia Schweppe*

## MIGRATION BIOGRAPHIES AND TRANSNATIONAL SOCIAL SUPPORT

This chapter focuses on forms and processes of transnational social support in the context of individual biographies of migration. The emphasis is on investigating what forms of transnational support become important at which moments and in which situations during the migration process; and what role they play in the migration process and in the life of a migrant. Thus, the relation between migration biographies and transnational social support is at the centre of this chapter.

To date, biographical analysis has generally been considered a less established approach in research on transnational support. Nevertheless, considering a transnational perspective on biographical developments of migrants is highly significant. In particular, we mention the research of Apitzsch (2003). Following Pries (2008) and Faist (2000b), Apitzsch takes up the concept of transnational space and presents the hypothesis that migration biographies can be described as the accumulated experiences of border crossings. Transnational space takes shape as the parameters and content of migration biographies are established and constantly reconstructed by the subjects of migration. Apitzsch understands biographies to be the locations in transnational space, defining *location* not in the sense of *topos* but in the sense of *topography* (Apitzsch 2003). Consequently, biographies in transnational space are not to be thought of as geographical locations but as invisible structures of state, legal, and cultural transitions interconnected in many ways. Individuals orient themselves in these structures and transitions through their individual biographies, and are collectively enmeshed with them at the same time. Biographies within migration processes as 'locations' within transnational spaces are to be understood as the intersection of collective structuration and individual construction. Consequently, according to Apitzsch and Siouti (2008), the study of transnational biographies is not about understanding biographies as a "product of subjectivity," but rather represents a methodological approach that explores the invisible but nevertheless objective structures of transnational migration spaces. These considerations open up new horizons to analyse the connections between migration biographies and transnational social support.

In general terms, social support refers to "the mechanisms through which a social environment protects individual members from threatening and impairing events and experiences and, in the event of those actually occurring, supports them in their efforts to cope"[1] (Nestmann 2001: 1687). Social support encompasses measures, interventions, and social relationships that help ease stressful and life-impairing events, situations, or processes (buffer effect). If there are no burdening influences, social support can also have a preventive function by promoting human well-being and welfare (direct effect). The concept of social support as it is used in this work does not limit support to "an active interplay between a focal person and his or her support network" (Vaux 1988: 29) but further encompasses the specific legal, institutional, and structural context within which people act. This allows us to focus on social processes and situate particular social supports within social and political contexts. It is an analysis that refers not only to coping with individual challenges, but also and particularly to the structural, organisational, and legal framing of scopes and limitations of action (cf. Homfeldt, Schröer, and Schweppe 2006).

In social support research people are considered as agents. With social structures changing, support structures will similarly become modified. Over time, they need to be re-built, actively negotiated, and constantly secured. Considered from a biographical perspective, this process takes place in the context of accumulated life experiences whereby social support also takes on a biographical dimension as it is shaped by the previous life history.

The special characteristic of transnational social support is its border-crossing nature. Transnational social support can be described as a social process of appropriating and constructing social worlds across national borders in which the social actors—migrants, in this case—develop, receive, accept, and provide transnational support within the social context of two or more countries in a direct or indirect manner (Homfeldt, Schröer, and Schweppe 2007). Following Apitzsch (2003), transnational social support therefore can be described as border-crossing experiences, which, from a biographical point of view, are reflected as accumulated experiences in migration biographies.

## THE CASE STUDY OF AMARÉ ISSAYU[2]

These considerations will be analysed in more detail within the following case study, which originates from a project investigating transnational ties of people with migration backgrounds living in Germany under precarious financial conditions. The research considers the importance of these ties for the life situation of the migrants. The following case analysis focuses on a partial aspect of the research in which we examine processes of transnational social support in the course of migration.

## METHODOLOGICAL APPROACH

In order to investigate the transnational ties of poor migrants, narrative-generating semi-structured interviews were conducted. Qualitative interviews provide the interviewees with an opportunity to express their world views and their experiences, thus making biographical experiences accessible to research. Qualitative interviews based on a narrative-generating approach are especially suitable to provide access to social reality from the perspective of the social actors, and to capture the many ways in which they experience social reality and how they are involved in creating it. As goals and motives are by no means always reflexively available to the actors involved, direct inquiries become almost impossible, and data collection by way of qualitative interviews proves to be a useful instrument. In the context of investigating transnational support processes within life-courses of migration, these interviews provide the opportunity not only to capture the subjective dimensions of these processes, but also to understand the structural conditions and the available scope of action within which support processes take place.

The interviews were conducted following the principle of theoretical sampling (Glaser and Strauss 1967), meaning that the first cases that were analysed generated a number of codes and categories that were later pursued through the selection of additional cases that could further illuminate this beginning conceptualisation. The interviews were audio-recorded and transcribed verbatim. Accordingly, dialects and slips of tongue have been considered.[3]

The analysis of the interviews was carried out according to the procedures of grounded theory as developed by Anselm Strauss (Strauss 1995). Initially, the transcripts of the interviews were interpreted line by line, followed by a comparative analysis aiming at a higher generalisation of concept development. In order to facilitate description and comprehension, this chapter explicitly refers to the case—contrary to the style of research usually used with grounded theory (which typically applies categories and codes abstracting from the case). Thus, the key categories and the relations identified in the course of the analysis are illuminated using the specific case.

## A BRIEF PROFILE OF AMARÉ ISSAYU

Our case study relates to the migration biography of Amaré Issayu. He grew up in an Ethiopian village and moved to Germany as a refugee in the early 1980s. Approximately six years later, his wife and their two children followed him to Germany. At the time of the interview, he was living in a small German town with his wife and four children. He worked as a warehouse employee and was fifty years old. In Ethiopia, Amaré Issayu completed a training programme in agriculture and worked in a government-run agricultural company. Due to very hard working conditions, particularly the intense heat when working in the fields, he worked there for only a short time. With the help of his relatives, he was given the opportunity to work as a teacher at a Catholic mission school, where he stayed for several years.

The political situation in Ethiopia was characterised by war, violence, and far-reaching restrictions on personal freedom.[4] He relates that at that time people were facing two alternatives: either take part in the war or be arrested. Amaré Issayu did not see any future for himself in Ethiopia and decided to migrate. The country of destination played only a secondary role in his migration process. The most important aspect for the social actor was 'to get out' of Ethiopia. Amaré Issayu made several attempts to leave the country legally but was confronted with a multitude of difficulties. The staff at the Italian, British, and Greek embassies that he approached frequently turned a deaf ear to his entreaties. He had to raise considerable funds, and experienced fraud and financial exploitation. For instance, his first attempt at leaving the country with an official letter of invitation to Italy failed as the letter was forged without his knowledge. He finally managed to provide the necessary money and migrated to Greece, although, given his limited funds, he could only migrate alone. His wife, who was pregnant at the time, and his two-year-old son remained in Ethiopia for the time being.

Amaré Issayu stayed in Greece for four months while looking for work. The search for work and an income are of significant importance in the process of migration. Amaré Issayu saw this as the only way to enable his wife and children to migrate as well. However, he was unable to find a suitable gainful employment in Greece and considered resuming the migration to move on to another country. He then made the acquaintance of a UN employee who opened up the prospect of migrating to Germany and helped him arrange all necessary formalities. With her help he obtained the permission to enter Germany.

Once in Germany, Amaré Issayu was first given accommodation in a refugee home. He describes his stay there as a horrible time, characterised by feelings of helplessness and powerlessness, characterised by heteronomy and a lack of options for action. He "*was taken*" from one refugee home to another, lived with other refugees in one small room without a shower, and worked for 1.50 euro per hour. Amaré Issayu says he had no choice but to submit to these living and working conditions and to endure them. The situation persisted for five years. Then new opportunities came up. The mayor of the town where Amaré Issayu lived at that time offered him a job as a cleaner in a warehouse. Even though he felt the work was degrading, disgraceful, and humiliating, he accepted it and still holds the same job today. His narrative reveals that he accepted both the experience of the refugee home and the humiliation of his work because he felt that this was the only way to have his family join him in Germany, given that regular work with a regular income is prerequisite to obtaining a German passport to ensure an uncomplicated entry into Germany for his family. Amaré Issayu was granted German citizenship in 1990, whereupon his wife and his two children were able to come to Germany.

## TRANSNATIONAL SOCIAL SUPPORT WITHIN THE PROCESS OF MIGRATION

The analysis of this case study shows that transnational social support took effect throughout Amaré Issayu's entire migration process. We will describe these moments alongside his migration biography.

### Transnational Organisation of Childcare within a Multi-generational Familial Care System

Shortly after his arrival in Greece, at the beginning of his migration process, Amaré Issayu received a letter from his wife informing him about the birth of their second child. Desperate, she let him know that she felt unable to care for and support both children and pleaded for help: "*The first child I cannot, I cannot, do all you can, I am not able to hold him.*" Amaré Issayu's migration has structural consequences upon the family caused by his physical absence as father and the loss of his income. In this situation, Amaré Issayu's wife felt unable to take on the role of sole caretaker and support both her children. However, Amaré Issayu's absence and the great geographical distance between them did not prevent her from involving him in finding a solution to the childcare problem.

Amaré Issayu was devastated when he received her letter: "*I locked my room and on the floor I really cry, cry, cry.*" His physical absence from his family prevented him from contributing directly to the problem's solution. Neither could he help by sending money since at the time (after his arrival in Greece) he lacked income from any gainful employment. However, he reacted to his wife's concern and her request for help as follows: "*So I send a letter back and I tell her, you can send my first child with my parents because my parents live 800 or 900 kilometers from the capital ( . . . ) and my brother, he live in the capital. I tell her, give the child to my brother, then he send it to my parents, they be happy when they see my kid.*"

He thus exercised the role and responsibility demanded by his wife from afar and came up with the suggestion for restructuring the family household to make sure that his children were being cared for. He resorted to a multi-generational family care system by proposing that his own parents take on the care of one of his children. Even the practical implementation of this decision was to be carried out within the family: Amaré Issayu relied on his brother to take his child to his grandparents, who lived 800 km away. Amaré Issayu's wife followed his suggestion and their older child was brought to live with the grandparents for the next six years, until the time when Amaré Issayu's wife and children could join him in Germany.

In describing these support structures, it became clear that their mobilisation did not require any negotiations. The narrative did not reveal any negotiations with the respective family members relating to whether, how, when, and for how long their support was needed. Neither the brother nor the parents were approached about the planned arrangement and asked for their consent. This suggests that support within the context of a three-generation family is a matter of course which is not altered by and does not become an issue due to the father's geographical distance. The 'naturalness' with which the support was provided also signifies its reliability. It is unconditional and can be activated at any time, for a short, medium, and even long period of time.

The support processes and structures just outlined can be described as a transnational organisation of childcare, put into effect within transnational family structures involving three generations. The transnational 'activation' of fatherhood by Amaré Issayu's wife is based on his initial response. He is able to influence the family structure in the country of origin at a distance and ensure care for his elder child. While his family's problems and the solution to the problem are communicated and organised transnationally, the implementation is carried out by local actors in the country of origin within the national or translocal context.

## 'Homelandmen' as Transnational Actors of Social Support

The initial phase of Amaré Issayu's migration process is not just characterised by alterations of the family structure in the country of origin and coping with challenges resulting from these changes, but is also shaped by the initial situations encountered upon arrival in the respective countries of destination—Greece and Germany—by the immigrant. During these phases 'homelandmen'—a word created by the social actor—are of central importance as transnational actors for providing support.

Amaré Issayu described the situation upon his arrival in Greece as follows: "*and had flown to Greece, and was at the airport in the Greece, I had no idea, no family, no people, nothing, I had no idea of hotel of the country ( . . . ), I was alone, no idea, everyone talking Greek, I don't talk Greek.*" His description dramatically illustrates the situation of feeling alien and his social disembeddedness from his surroundings. After a short time at the airport he decided to take a taxi to go into town. Halfway to the city, however, he asked the driver to take him back to the airport since he did not trust the driver who wanted to take him to a specific hotel. The taxi driver dropped him off at a small hostel close to the airport where Amaré Issayu stayed for one week until he realised that he was running out of money. After a few days, he told the landlady that he had no money left and had to go to the city to look for 'homelandmen.' This is the first indication that the search for 'homelandmen' is connected with the search for support in a situation where new means of action are required in order to continue the migration process. This also shows that Amaré Issayu anticipated the presence of 'homelandmen' in a special place: *the city*.

His landlady offered him free accommodation in exchange for helping her clean the rooms and prepare breakfast. After one month, Amaré Issayu realised that although his time there was enjoyable, he had to leave to search for 'homelandmen' in the city, or otherwise look for opportunities to migrate to other countries. The work he was doing was not what Amaré Issayu considered to be a long-term possibility. Therefore, meeting 'homelandmen' or continuing the migration process to another country were perceived as options to improve his situation.

Amaré Issayu made several attempts to obtain an entry visa to Italy in order to migrate from there to the United States. During this time, Amaré Issayu shared a small basement apartment with four other refugees. After a while, he met a UN employee who made it possible for him to obtain an entry visa to Germany. By opening up new opportunities to migrate—opportunities that Amaré Issayu deemed to be very viable for his future—this staff person came to be of great importance in his migration process. Migrating to Germany meant for him the possibility of improving his life situation, mainly by obtaining more opportunities for gainful employment.

In his narrative, it stands out that in contrast to the housemates who are not described in great detail, Amaré Issayu introduces the UN employee and describes her as having grown up in Greece but having "*black skin as I have*" and being from Ethiopia. This is the first time in his narrative that Amaré Issayu meets someone who comes close to what he refers to as a 'homelandman.' Both her skin color and her country of origin are decisive points of reference. The person who eventually enables him to migrate shares two critical attributes with Amaré Issayu—coming from Ethiopia and having, as Amaré Issayu repeatedly points out, black skin. However, when describing the woman, distinguishing marks seem to set her apart her from a 'homelandman': even though the woman is originally from Ethiopia, she grew up in Greece. Another distinguishing mark for the respondent is her gender, a fact which also prevents her from being a 'homeland*man*.'

After initiating the second part of the migration with the help of this woman, Amaré Issayu arrived in Germany, where he intended to apply for asylum. Back in Greece, a friend of his had given him the address of a person living in Germany. Amaré Issayu tried to contact this person immediately upon his arrival, but his repeated attempts proved futile. The social actor again feels all alone but it is only for a brief moment that he does not know what to do. He starts wandering the streets of the German town in order to find a 'homelandman.' The search for 'homelandmen' is initiated in a situation similar to the one in Greece described earlier, when the strategy to deal with the situation he encounters upon arrival proves ineffective. The search for 'homelandmen' is consistently conducted in a context where new options are required to continue the migration process.

Considering that Amaré Issayu does not know any 'homelandmen' and has no addresses indicating where they might be found, the question arises of how he looks for them and manages to find them. His strategy, described by the actor as *"walking around the city and looking for a homelandman,"* follows the criteria just described: First of all, the skin color is an identifying mark which enables him to recognise potential 'homelandmen.' Since not every person with dark skin is from Ethiopia, and the skin color in itself is not a sufficient distinguishing mark to identify a compatriot, language is the second essential criterion. Amaré Issayu seeks out black men in the streets and starts talking to them in his mother tongue. If the person he addresses understands him and responds, Amaré Issayu can be certain that he has met a 'homelandman.' Language and skin color are the identifying marks enabling Amaré Issayu to recognise compatriots. These two features become the symbols of the country of origin these individuals have in common.

After walking the streets of the German town for a while, Amaré Issayu actually found a 'homelandman.' He explained to him his situation and mentioned that he had just arrived in Germany and had been unable to meet his sole contact person. Amaré Issayu asked his compatriot: *"What can I do now?"* and received the answer: *"Come with me."* Subsequently, Amaré Issayu received the help and support he needed: he was able to sleep at the home of his compatriot, who accompanied him the following day to the authorities where he applied for asylum. He could also leave his money and passport at this person's house for safekeeping over several weeks. The support he hoped to receive from his compatriots was effectively provided. This man enabled him to initiate the next steps of his migration process.

Against the background of these situations, the support system provided by 'homelandmen' can be described in greater detail. Amaré Issayu hoped to receive support based on a person belonging to a certain group of people. Indeed, they actually responded to this expectation. The correspondence between expected and provided support is a central prerequisite for the viability of this support system. The analysis also shows that being personally acquainted with someone is not a necessary condition for the activation of this support system. A long relationship or previous interactions are not necessary in order to expect and receive support. The support system is rather constituted by an imagined community whose members belong to it due to certain ascriptive features.[5] Apart from country of origin, they have in common a shared skin color and mother tongue, indicators that the same migration history comes into play. 'Homelandmen' are persons who have made the same decision, to leave their common country of origin—Ethiopia—in order to migrate to the same country of destination. The structure of relationships within this support system is characterised by the fact that the supporting party does not expect anything in return, at least not immediately. Relationships seem to be short-term and focused on the purpose of support. Trust is another discernible factor, manifested in the fact that Amaré Issayu felt trusting enough to leave his passport and his money with a hitherto unknown compatriot.

What is essential within this support system is not only that support is provided. It is provided effectively. Difficulties created by the initial situation upon arrival were overcome and Amaré Issayu was able to continue his migration process. The decisive factor for this was the migration history the actors shared in common, although their experiences occurred at different time periods. Their earlier migration had provided Amaré Issayu's compatriots with knowledge and experience regarding the circumstances of life in the respective countries. He also drew on their familiarity with the regulations of the migration process in Germany, including paperwork and administrative formalities. It is precisely this kind of knowledge that was important for Amaré Issayu to orient himself in an environment that was alien to him in order to be able to continue his migration.

Ultimately, 'homelandmen' represent a support system that exactly fits Amaré Issayu's needs in dealing with the initial difficulties upon arrival in the countries of destination. In an alien environment, not knowing anyone and lacking country-specific knowledge to orient himself, Amaré Issayu connects with something familiar based on the common country of origin and migration course. He thus constitutes an imaginary group of people, to whom he belongs and whom he trusts. His need for support is met and an appropriate and effective response is made possible based on the previously acquired knowledge and experience of his compatriots. Figuratively speaking, 'homelandmen' take on the job of a 'translator' or a 'guide,' helping him to translate the strangeness around him into something that is understandable, to help him find his way. Consequently, 'homelandmen' represent a transnational link for Amaré Issayu. By establishing contact with something familiar from his home country he is given access to the new and unfamiliar countries of destination.

## "You always have to help"—the Ambivalence of Financial Remittances

Another form of transnational support is the financial support Amaré Issayu provides for his family in Ethiopia. He did not support his family from the beginning of his migration, but was able to do so only once his situation in Germany had become more or less stable: namely once he had obtained German citizenship, had found work, and had his wife and children follow him to Germany.

Amaré Issayu understands financial support as an obligation: "*We have to help because we grew up there and we know the problems people face.*" As such, the obligation to help is a commitment and duty for all those who have grown up in Ethiopia and have experienced the problematic conditions of life. The obligation to help is also closely linked to his religious socialisation in Ethiopia: "*Religion, when you grow into a religion from when you are a child, and Christ says every Sunday to 'help' and 'do it well' or, like what the priest say from when you are a child until now, it is always inside.*" Amaré Issayu describes the obligation to help as a norm that is internalised ("*is inside*"), deeply rooted in his biography, and still present in his life today ("*until now*"). The norm is independent of location and maintains its validity also in Germany.

The norm of having to help is of particular importance within a family and even more so in the intergenerational relationship with his parents. Amaré Issayu recounts in detail the efforts, struggles, and sacrifices his parents have made under precarious living conditions to give their six children a good education and secure a better life for them. In return, Amaré Issayu feels it is his "duty" to help his parents now that he is an adult: "*That is duty, because the parents done everything for us there, and now we have better chances, for example go to Europe, house, shower, car.*" Their efforts place the children under an obligation to help and tie the generations together.

However, the narration also reveals his ambivalence regarding his religious socialisation and the related obligation to help. Amaré Issayu says: "*Religion is often suffocating.*" "Suffocating" can be understood in the sense of a threat for one's own life and existence. The following quotation points out the "suffocating" quality of this obligation: "*I want a lot, I want save money, I want luxury like the others, but on my back there is a burden, I cannot do this, because half my life is 25 years, now half my life is there and here and I live well (.) I say it no matter if you're on welfare.*" Against the background of precarious financial means, the dilemma of having to help results from the desire to improve his own material situation in order to achieve a standard of living similar to that of other people in Germany and to participate in the country's wealth while, at the same time, having to provide financial support to his family. When Amaré Issayu says that half of his life he spent in Ethiopia and the other half in Germany, he places himself in two systems of reference which both demand the improvement of material living conditions. Due to the scarce resources he has at his disposal, these demands can hardly be satisfied simultaneously. In this situation he opts to provide financial support to his family in Ethiopia, a choice that necessarily entails limitations to the improvement of his own life in Germany. Therefore, the "suffocating" character of the obligation to help can be interpreted as a limitation to the improvement of his own material living conditions in Germany. His statement: "*I live well, I say it no matter if you're on welfare*" may be seen as an attempt to deal with this conflict by rating his living conditions as "*good*" and qualifying the meaning of potential dependence on social benefits.[6]

At irregular intervals Amaré Issayu sends money to his parents, sometimes 50 euros, sometimes less. He says: "*There ( . . . ) 50 euro is a lot of money for them, can buy something, clothes, food, maybe it's not 'nough but they have the hope 'look, our child has grown up better, become more an adult ( . . . ) now he also thinks for us'.*" It is obvious that he emphasises the amount he gives and the contribution it makes to the family's livelihood in Ethiopia, while simultaneously expressing doubts regarding the adequacy of the sum ("*maybe it's not 'nough*"). Doubting the adequacy of the remittances is bound to imply doubting the fulfillment of his obligation to help, because he has to not only help, but also provide 'good help' as the foregoing quotation indicates ("*help and do it well*"). The obligation to help thus does not only generate the conflict of wanting to improve his own and his parents' living conditions at the same time. In addition, he is also confronted with the question of whether the help he provides is appropriate and as such "good" and whether he lives up to the expectations beyond the mere provision of money. When Amaré Issayu then says that even if the money he sends may help his parents keep up the hope that their son has "*grown up better*" and is "*more adult,*" he not only attributes a material value to his money transfers but also emphasises their emotional value. In accordance with their efforts to enable their son to have a "good" and—compared to themselves—better life, the remittances will give his parents the impression that their son is doing well. In addition, Amaré Issayu says that the money transfers also show that "*now he also thinks for us.*" Remittances as a sign of "thinking *for* the parents" refer to the son taking responsibility for his parents. In an analogy to the responsibility taken for the aging generation, as indicated earlier, Amaré Issayu can demonstrate his concern for his aging parents. The immaterial functions he attributes to his remittances can thus be interpreted as Amaré Issayu's attempt to counteract his doubts about the adequacy of his help.

## Transnational Aging in Ethiopia

One day, Amaré Issayu wishes to return to Ethiopia to live there. His desire to return is closely linked to his idea of "home." Amaré Issayu says: "*No matter where you are, home is home.*" It becomes clear that home is irrevocable; home is unalterable. Amaré Issayu assumes that home is the place "*where you were born, grow up.*" The time from birth to young adulthood defines where home is. For Amaré Issayu, home is closely linked to language and to culture: "*home is the language, the culture.*" Consequently, home is not so much defined by people or interpersonal relationships, but rather by the place of growing up, by learning to speak the respective language, and by being familiar with a certain culture. In his opinion, even long-time experience in other countries does not change the fact that home is where a person has grown up: "*You can be in the society or in the culture and the language and you must join in, but that doesn't change your home, your home language or your home sickness, I just want to say 95 percent you don't change where your home is.*" He assumes that this understanding of home is universally valid. He believes that people ultimately wish to return to their origins, no matter whether their migration is regional or international, as evidenced in this statement: "*I see many people, I hear, home is home, for example also in Germany from German people I hear this home is home, I go home, say just you come here from Bavaria to work, to live, in the end when you retire, you go back, with your relatives, your friends, my opinion is it no matter where you go, home is home.*" Later Amaré Issayu says: "*Abroad you are always foreign, a foreigner, is always foreigner.*" The question arises to what extent his understanding of home can also be seen as a reaction to specific experiences in Germany. Being a foreigner points to experiences of difference, of being different, and of not belonging, while home stands for familiarity and belonging. The wording "*you are always a foreigner*" (and not "it is foreign to me") points to interactive processes whereby this foreignness is either created or attributed by others. He is given the status of a foreigner by others, and is made a foreigner in comparison with others. Returning to the home country can also be understood as the search for familiarity and a sense of belonging as well as a desire to end the feeling of being different and not belonging. The universal nature of his statement that abroad a foreigner will always remain a foreigner safely suggests that he believes this experience of difference is not just an individual problem affecting only him.[7]

The time of his return to Ethiopia depends on two different factors. The first is related to the time of his retirement and to receiving the old-age pension which he needs for his livelihood in Ethiopia. For economic reasons, he rules out returning at the current time: "*The problem is what can I take now, how can I live there when I go back, but how can I go back now, what have I in my hands, what have I in the future if I go back, I am in the streets there and have no money there, how can I do that, not possible.*" Consequently, the time of his return is tied to his work in Germany and to the German pension system.

The second factor is related to the time when his children will be able to take care of themselves and live independent lives. In accordance with his understanding of home, Amaré Issayu sees his children's future in Germany. The children have grown up in Germany; consequently, he considers Germany their home: "*Children for example ( . . . ), for them you can say I am born here, I am German, I stay there.*" What are the consequences of the different perspectives that Amaré Issayu sees for himself and anticipates for his children? He accepts the anticipated future perspective for his children. He wishes to stay with them in Germany until they are able to take care of themselves. Amaré Issayu tries very hard to get his children onto a "*good track*" with this aim in mind. He explains that this duty results from the experience he has had with his own parents.

For the spatial separation that will follow his return to Ethiopia, Amaré Issayu has designed a relational model that is almost identical to his current relationship he has with his own parents: "*When I go home, my children come visit, or maybe help when I have no money, maybe as said before 10 euro or 50 euro per month, too.*" The desire to see his children come to Ethiopia and the hope placed on their support of him in cases of financial emergency imply his wish for a biographical continuity of the current transnational relationships he takes part in between family generations. Just as he has experienced his parents' struggle and concern to enable him to have a comparatively better life, in turn he expects his children to support their parents during old age. The concern and support for the aging father are to be provided transnationally, just as Amaré Issayu is now providing his support. The question remains, however, to what extent this generational model may change when the father receives a pension and can rely on an income, albeit a potentially small one. Ultimately, Amaré Issayu designs a retirement model for himself that can be called 'transnational age(ing) at home'—aging at home has its financial basis in the working life spent in Germany and the subsequent pension arrangement, and is shaped by transnational relationships between family generations.

## TRANSNATIONAL FAMILY CARE AND THE SOLIDARY-BASED COMMUNITY OF 'HOMELANDMEN'

The case study of Amaré Issayu illustrates that, depending on the stages of the migration process, different forms of support become relevant and different actors fulfill different functions. In this context, support systems consisting of family members or compatriots are of particular importance. With respect to these two support systems, the analysis showed and confirmed the naturalness with which support is expected, provided, and received. There are no negotiations about whether, in which way, and at what time support is to be provided.

## THE FAMILIAL SUPPORT SYSTEM IN A TRANSNATIONAL CONTEXT

Transnational support processes in a family context play a key role throughout the entire migration process. Transnational family support takes place in the context of three family generations. The actors involved provide support as well as receive it. They take over different support functions depending on their respective phases in life. For instance, the grandparents appear as actors providing support with the upbringing of their grandchildren in response to the care problem caused by the father's migration. In exchange, the generation of adult children (son) provides material support to the grandparents. At the same time, the generation of adult children is also responsible for the upbringing of the younger generation of grandchildren, be it in the country of origin while they still remain there or in the country of destination. For instance, the mother communicates her concern about the children caused by the absence of the father by way of a 'transnational call for help,' upon the receipt of which the father organises and arranges care through the grandparents transnationally. Once the children have arrived in the destination country the parents take over the childcare.

Existing research on social support along with the results of transnational family research offers explanations for these findings. At a national level, social support research has repeatedly confirmed the family to be a reliable, important, and constant source of support (e.g., Pierce, Sarason, and Sarason 1996). The main reason is the special quantity and quality of familial and kin support due to norms of family solidarity. Family solidarity—as shown by transnational family research—does not vanish due to geographical distance (e.g., Goulbourne and Chamberlain 2001; Herrera Lima 2001; Bryceson and Vuorela 2002; de la Hoz 2004; Pribilsky 2004). It forms the basis of providing support to family members equally at a transnational level.

Within research on transnational family support, the support between parents and children, in particular between mothers and children, has been extensively investigated, with special attention being paid to the phenomenon of transnational motherhood (e.g., Bernhard, Landolt, and Goldring 2005; Hondagneu-Sotelo and Avila 1997; Lutz 2007). The case of Amaré Issayu points to the importance of 'transnational fatherhood' which may accompany the activation of intergenerational transnational and national support systems. In this study, it became apparent that the absent father, despite his physical distance, was actively included in organising the childcare, and that the activation of fatherhood and its border-crossing implementation are part of a complex interaction of the family support activities as a whole. Furthermore, the case study of Amaré Issayu shows the importance of including the generation of the grandparents (and possibly other family members) in further research on transnational family care.

Also of relevance for future transnational research on familial support are the indications occurring in this case of the burdens, ambivalences, and difficulties faced by the middle generation in regard to the financial support for family members in the country of origin, especially when provided or asked to be provided under conditions of poverty or in financially precarious life situations. Under these conditions, solidarity norms and their observance or even compliance may be burdensome, and can generate considerable pressure. This expectation may deteriorate the quality of life of the supporters due to additional financial burdens, limiting the satisfaction of their own needs or the needs of the family living in Germany. In particular, tensions may arise with respect to familial and generational distributive justice (Hollstein, Huber, and Schweppe 2009). In order not to overlook such burdensome, restrictive, or negative consequences, the present focus on migrants contributing to overcoming poverty in their countries of origin should be expanded by looking at the actors providing support. Migrant remittances are becoming increasingly relevant in international politics to combat poverty in the countries of origin and have been made the object of numerous private and public programmes in order to promote their development potential. Against this background, the proposed research perspective is of particular relevance (cf. Schweppe 2011).

## THE SOLIDARY COMMUNITY OF THE 'HOMELANDMEN'

With respect to the support system of 'homelandmen,' a parallel based on principles of solidarity becomes apparent. These principles are based on criteria other than those within the family. In the context of the support relationships among compatriots, it is not necessary to be closely acquainted or to know each other personally in order to receive or give support. The fact that compatriots are concerned seems to be sufficient in order to (naturally) provide support for people in the same country of destination, and for those who are in need of it to accept it. According to what has been outlined, possible explanations for this phenomenon are closely related to the similarities in country of origin and migration history, commonality in skin color and language, along with shared representations of a solidarity-based community. Consequently, compatriot support appears to be built on the basis of a shared biographical background along with the related experiences from which closeness and mutual trust develop.

In order to further explain the support system of 'homelandmen,' reference can be made to the discussions on transnational communities in the research on transnationalism. Certainly, despite a broad discussion on the concept of transnational community, this concept still remains unclear and has taken on a variety of meanings. In general, transnational communities develop on the basis of specific social, cultural, political, and/or economic interests and motivations, common regional and/or national origin, or common values or ideologies, and on the transnational behaviour of the people involved. Faist assumes that these communities, which are not based on kinship, do not require their members to live in two or more countries at the same time, but the decisive factor is "that communities without propinquity link through exchange, reciprocity, and solidarity to achieve a high degree of social cohesion, and a common repertoire of symbolic and cultural representations" (Faist, quoted in Sökefeld 2008: 214).

Following these considerations, Sökefeld (2008) assumes that diaspora can be described as a subtype of transnational communities. The diaspora differs from other transnational communities by the fact that its transnational relations, being its constituting features, are mainly of a cultural (i.e., symbolic) kind, and that these symbolic relationships are not necessarily based on transnational social relationships established through direct interactions. Accordingly, he understands diaspora as follows:

Diaspora can be defined then as a transnational imagined community that is based on an identity that is territorially related but not limited to the place in which the members of the diaspora live. ( . . . ) Significant ( . . . ) is the idea of a shared identity and a sentiment of solidarity that is implied in the imagination of community. That is, the members of the community take interest in the lives of those that are imagined as fellow members of the community elsewhere. Yet this interest and solidarity need not take the particular shape of a sentiment of home and origin that is projected on this elsewhere (Sökefeld 2008: 218).

In transferring these considerations to the case of Amaré Issayu, the support system of compatriots can be explained in more detail. According to Amaré Issayu's imagination, 'homelandmen' are members of a community whose binding element is the common country of origin, which the members did not leave, in most cases, as refugees. Connected with this community is the idea of solidarity among its members, for otherwise he would not turn to them in situations where he needs support. Because of his own migration path, Amaré Issayu meets the criteria to be granted access to this community and to become part of it. The imagined community proves real to the extent that his need for support is met. In the case of Amaré Issayu, the potential for solidarity of the community finds its expression in forms and processes of social support during the initial situation in the country of arrival. The idea of a solidarity-based community is the answer to the question of why Amaré Issayu does not need to know the individual compatriots personally. Ultimately, 'homelandmen' are depersonalised representatives of an (imagined) solidarity-based community. As individuals they are (only) important to the extent that they provide access to and enact the solidarity potential in the community.[8] Apart from solidarity, trust becomes apparent as another element which characterises the direct relationships among its members in the context of providing and receiving social support.

As a result, the connection between transnational communities and social support, with respect to diasporic transnational communities, proves to be of relevance for future transnational support research. Until now social support processes within transnational communities have hardly been investigated systematically. In this context the concept of moral economy of the diaspora developed by Radtke and Schlichte (2004) may be useful.

Moral economies are based on an imagined community. With respect to the moral economy of people in exile, Radtke and Schlichte (2004) assume that these communities, similar to what we have argued, are formed on the basis of a shared language, an identical fate, and the experiences encountered in exile. Moral economies can be considered exchange systems whose central exchange partners are not necessarily individuals, as is the case in personal relationships. Instead, the individual is perceived as a member of a greater community, beyond the reciprocal relationships of kinship and family. If these exchange relationships are based on moral demands, which take on both a material and an immaterial character, consolidate, and become a complex structure, the resulting process can be thought of as a moral economy. Communities of this kind extending beyond territorial borders are described as 'transnational moral economies.' The moral economy in exile, according to Radtke and Schlichte (2004: 184), consists of "differentiated systems of giving and obligations, for instance support in finding work and accommodation, provision of clothes, accommodation and food during short-term transition periods," which contribute mainly to "dealing with the uncertainty during the first phase of exile."[9] The authors assume that the moral economy is established through the exchange "of small services" and "few goods" because personal bonds are formed and reproduced during the extended period between giving and receiving in return. "Because giving, receiving and returning are not required to take place in direct succession, the time difference between meeting these obligations spans the relationships between those performing the exchange" (Radtke and Schlichte 2004: 184).[10] Relationships between the exchanging parties form and consolidate over time especially because the support requires something in return which, however, must not be given immediately. Subtle forms of social control are employed to make sure that the obligation to give something in return is met. This informal system of sanctions would take effect due to the fear of loss of face by "allocation of honor and shame" (Radtke and Schlichte 2004: 184). This in turn implies "the 'publicity' of an imagined or real community" (Radtke and Schlichte 2004: 185).[11]

According to this model, social support within transnational diasporic communities could be described as exchange relationships expressed via the triad of giving, receiving, and returning (cf. Mauss 1989). In the case of Amaré Issayu, however, no statement can be made as to the extent of his obligation to return the received and accepted social support from members of the community, and whether he will be subjected to mechanisms of social control in case he gives nothing in return. Neither are there any indications of the assumed forming of relationships between the exchanging persons in the period of receiving support and the point of returning it. Our data rather point to a short-term relationship with the respective supporters, limited to the period of receiving the support. However, it might be possible that by receiving support Amaré Issayu enters into a commitment towards the community. That is, it would not be necessary to immediately give something in return to the persons who actually provided the support, but he would become a member of the community and enter into a commitment of solidarity towards this collective.

Finally it is important to retain that 'homelandmen' are the ones whom the newly arrived turn to as a first instance and they facilitate the initial phase in the country of destination, particularly when other sources of support, such as established social services, are not used. However, the support system of compatriots is inasmuch restricted as it depends on their presence and their actual encounters.

## CONCLUSION AND PERSPECTIVE

Since both support systems, 'homelandmen' and family, can be related to concepts of solidarity, there is an affinity between them. This affinity becomes apparent through the importance of the reliability of support and the familiarity of the support partners. While within the support system of compatriots the relationship is built on an imagined solidarity-based community to which support functions are attributed due to common characteristics (skin color, language, upbringing in the country of origin, migration history), the reliability in familial support systems is based on norms of obligation originating from intergenerational moral concepts and religious values. A parallel exists in that both family transnational support and closeness to 'homelandmen' are based on biographic experiences made in the country of origin and both are explained by an early socialisation linked to the same location. And local support by compatriots in the country of arrival is transnational to the extent that this support system is based on experiences and knowledge acquired in both the country of origin and the country of destination. Consequently, investigating the relation between migration biographies and transnational social support proves to be insightful as it reveals the complex interaction between both. Following Apitzsch (2003), migration biographies reveal invisible but nevertheless objective structures of transnational migration spaces, and reflect the transnational support processes, which in turn are reflected in and simultaneously shaped by individual biographies.

## NOTES

1. Translation from German by the authors.
2. The names of the persons discussed in this case have been modified to ensure their anonymity.
3. Due to the translation of the interviews, which were conducted in German, the literal transcription has partly been lost as have the interviewees' dialects, grammatical mistakes, and slips of tongue.
4. At that time there were a number of armed conflicts in Ethiopia. In 1975 the so-called 'Second Ogaden War' started between Ethiopia and Somalia. It only ended in 1984. In addition, several resistance groups within the country started armed struggles against the central government. The 'Tigray conflict' lasted from 1975 until 1991, and the 'Oromo conflict' from 1976 to 1993 (http://www.sozialwiss.uni-hamburg.de/onTEAM/preview/Ipw/Akuf/archiv_afrika.htm, access date: June 2, 2011).
5. Using the example of nations, Benedict Anderson characterises imagined communities as communities whose members "will never know most of their fellow-members, meet them or even hear oft them, yet in the minds of each lives the image of their communion" (Anderson 2006: 6). In this regard he asserts that "in fact, all communities larger than primordial villages of face-to-face contact (and perhaps even these) are imagined. As a second characteristic of imagined communities he mentions that they are "conceived as a deep, horizontal comradeship" (Anderson 2006: 7).

6. The fact that he qualifies the importance of money is also evident in the following statement: "*I cannot save money but (.) if my mother would be ill or when she would die or if my sister will be concerned with something, what is the use of money for me then? I love my sister or my mother live.*"
7. Amaré Issayu develops different practices to create his Ethiopian home in Germany. For instance, he meets up with other people from Ethiopia in order to hold special coffee ceremonies he has known in Ethiopia when he was an adolescent. By maintaining those ceremonies, the smells and aromas make him feel as if he were back in Ethiopia. Amaré Issayu feels very much at ease then. Also other "*things from home*" (for instance, specially prepared meals and traditional clothes) achieve this goal.
8. This corresponds to the concepts of generalised reciprocity and diffuse solidarity as it is used by Faist (2000a). "Generalized reciprocity means that the equivalence of exchange between actors is not exactly determined. This implies that the exchanging partners are not considered specific persons but rather as members of a bigger group such as a member of a village, a religious community or a nation. The concept of multiple reciprocity is helpful for further explanation. While specific reciprocity demands a bilateral equilibrium between clearly defined agents, in case of generalized reciprocity it is a balance within the group which is important" (Faist 2000a: 37f).
9. Translation from German by the authors.
10. Translation from German by the authors.
11. Translation from German by the authors.

## BIBLIOGRAPHY

Anderson, B. (2006) *Imagined Communities. Reflections on the Origin and Spread of Nationalism*. London and New York: Verso.
Apitzsch, U. (2003) 'Migrationsbiographien als Orte transnationaler Räume.' In *Migration, Biographie und Geschlechterverhältnisse*, edited by U. Apitzsch and M. M. Jansen, 65–80. Münster: Westfälisches Dampfboot.
Apitzsch, U., and I. Siouti (2008) 'Transnationale Biographien.' In *Soziale Arbeit und Transnationalität*, edited by H. G. Homfeldt, W. Schröer, and C. Schweppe, 97–111. Weinheim and München: Juventa.
Bernhard, J. K., P. Landolt, and L. Goldring (2005) 'Transnational, Multi-Local Motherhood: Experiences of Separation and Reunification among Latin American Families in Canada.' *Early Childhood Education Publications and Research*. Paper 6, http://digitalcommons.ryerson.ca/cgi/viewcontent.cgi?article=1005&context=ece (accessed May 24, 2011).
Bryceson, D., and U. Vuorela (2002) *The Transnational Family. New European Frontiers and Global Networks*. Oxford and New York: Berg.
de la Hoz, P. F. (2004) 'Familienleben, Transnationalität und Diaspora.' *ÖIF Materialien 21*, http://www.oif.ac.at/aktuell/MAT21_Familienleben_Diaspora_2004.pdf .
Faist, T. (2000a) 'Grenzen überschreiten. Das Konzept Transstaatliche Räume und seine Anwendungen.' In *Transstaatliche Räume: Politik, Wirtschaft und Kultur in und zwischen Deutschland und der Türkei*, edited by T. Faist, 9–56. Bielefeld: Transcript.
Faist, T. (2000b) *The Volume and Dynamics of International Migration and Transnational Social Spaces*. Oxford: Oxford University Press.
Glaser, B. G., and A. L. Strauss (1967) *The Discovery of Grounded Theory: Strategies for Qualitative Research*. Chicago: Aldine Publishing Company.
Goulbourne, H., and M. Chamberlain, eds. (2001) *Caribbean Families in Britain and the Trans-Atlantic World*. London: Macmillan.

Herrera Lima, F. (2001) 'Transnational Families: Institutions of Transnational Social Spaces.' In *New Transnational Social Spaces. International Migration and Transnational Companies in the Early Twenty-First Century*, edited by L. Pries, 77–92. London: Routledge.

Hollstein, T., L. Huber, and C. Schweppe (2009) 'Transmigration und Arrmut. Zwischen prekärer Unterstützung und risikohafter Bewältigung.' *Zeitschrift für Sozialpädagogik*, 4: 360–72.

Homfeldt, H. G., W. Schröer, and C. Schweppe (2006) *Transnationalität, soziale Unterstützung, agency*. Nordhausen: Traugott Bautz.

Homfeldt, H. G., W. Schröer, and C. Schweppe (2007) 'Transnationalisierung Sozialer Arbeit. Transmigration, soziale Unterstützung und Agency.' *Neue Praxis*, 3: 239–49.

Hondagneu-Sotelo, P., and E. Avila (1997) "'I'm Here, but I'm There': The Meaning of Latina Transnational Motherhood.' *Gender and Society*, 11(5): 548–71.

Lutz, H. (2007) *Vom Weltmarkt in den Privathaushalt: Die neuen Dienstmädchen im Zeitalter der Globalisierung*. Opladen: Barbara Budrich.

Mauss, M. (1989) 'Die Gabe. Form und Funktion des Austauschs in archaischen Gesellschaften.' In *Soziologie und Anthropologie*. Vol. 2, edited by M. Mauss, 9–144. Frankfurt a. M.: Suhrkamp.

Nestmann, F. (2001) 'Soziale Netzwerke—Soziale Unterstützung.' In *Handbuch Sozialarbeit/Sozialpädagogik*, edited by H.-U. Otto and H. Thiersch, 1684–93. Neuwied: Luchterhand.

Pierce, G. R., B. R. Sarason, and I. G. Sarason, eds. (1996) *Handbook of Social Support and the Family*. New York: Plenum Press.

Pribilsky, J. (2004) "'Aprendemos a convivir': Conjugal Relations, Co-parenting, and Family Life among Ecuadorian Transnational Migrants in New York City and the Ecuadorian Andes.' *Global Networks*, 4(3): 313–34.

Pries, L. (2008) *Die Transnationalisierung der sozialen Welt*. Frankfurt a.M.: Suhrkamp.

Radtke, K., and K. Schlichte (2004) 'Bewaffnete Gruppen und die moralische Ökonomie der Diaspora.' In *Transnationale Solidarität. Chancen und Grenzen*, edited by J. Beckert, J. Eckert, M. Kohli, and W. Streeck, 181–94. Frankfurt a.M.: Campus.

Schweppe, C. (2011) Migrant Financial Remittances—Between Development Policy and Transnational Family Care". *Transnational Social Review—A Social Work Journal*, 1:39–53.

Sökefeld, M. (2008) *Struggling for Recognition: The Alevi in Germany and in Transnational Space*. New York: Berghahn Books.

Strauss, A. L. (1995) *Grundlagen qualitativer Sozialforschung. Datenanalyse und Theoriebildung in der empirischen und soziologischen Forschung*. München: W. Fink.

Vaux, A. (1988) *Social Support: Theory, Research and Intervention*. New York: Praeger.

# 9 Transnational Biographies
## The Delimitation of Motherhood

*Elisabeth Tuider*

"Identities [free themselves] of particular points in time, places,
pasts and traditions—
they are delivered and appear free-floating."

(Hall 1994: 212)

The 'deterritorialisation' of economic and social connections, a 'com-
pression' of space and time as well as a 'delimitation' of the lifeworld are
part of the contemporary social scientific vocabulary, since, as a result
of globalisation and migration, it seemed that societies have lost their
nation-state identities in favour of a polyphonous character. Corresponding to this societal diagnosis, identities are also being conceived of as
liquefied and decentralised. At the level of the individual, a "transnational spatial polygamy" (Beck 1997) can be observed, and life plans
and forms of living that were previously localised are today being trans-
ported by the media throughout the entire world in the form of imagina-
tions (Appadurai 1991).

With the delimitation of the lifeworld, however, as I would like to propose here, life plans are not necessarily being decoupled from specific
resources. This means that even in a spatially polygamous world, access to
resources (such as residence status, age, or gender) remains important for
the social behaviour of people. Identities and biographies only *appear* there
to be free-floating, as Hall (1994) has suggested to us in the opening quotation. The constitution of a person's identity and biography is influenced by
intersectionally entangled power relationships as well as by new, transnational conditions of exploitation.

The simultaneity of delimitation and limitation is taken up in this chapter, and from this perspective the relationship between transnationalisation and biography is defined in more detail. Against the backdrop of the
theoretical considerations that have been briefly articulated so far, I devote
the following chapter to the repercussions that spatial, migration-related
distance has on the family's system of relationships and the situation of
women in the family, as well as on the way in which it shapes motherhood.
By what actual practices do migrated women maintain an active motherhood in relation to their children in the region of origin and, in doing so,
how do they establish continuity, closeness, and care? Does this lead to the

development of new forms of motherhood or, quite the reverse, does it lead to a negation of motherhood (cf. Nobles 2006)?

I also investigate the thesis that new forms and practices of mothering emerge in (transnational) migration spaces. The Mexican-U.S.-American border region serves as a point of departure for understanding delimited biographies.[1] Using the case study of biographical stories[2] of women *maquiladora* labourers[3] who live in Ciudad Juárez and are originally from Durango in Mexico, I illustrate the new challenges facing motherhood in transnational spaces. In doing so, my fundamental assumption is that a migration-related delimitation of motherhood does occur, but not its disintegration.

## TRANSMIGRATION AND BIOGRAPHY

During the beginnings of transnationalisation research and under the influence of (economic) globalisation debates, transnationality was analysed under the perspective through which products and capital, technological achievements and knowledge, as well as labourers and services are exchanged and mobilised (Faist 2007). As an extension of this analytic perspective, eventually social research focused on the social practices by which human beings shape and arrange their migration-related, delimited lifeworlds.

The transmigration research[4] that has arisen since the 1990s attends to the economic, social, cultural, and political connections that migrants maintain with their country of origin (cf. Basch, Glick Schiller, and Blanc-Szanton 1994). Alongside the forms of migration that had been discussed up to that point—immigration, return migration, and diaspora—from the end of the twentieth century a growing form of migration has been identified: transmigration. Transmigration is characterised by commuting between different geographical, national, and cultural spaces.

Migration flows from the 'global South' have elicited altered perspectives, especially in gender research and in migration research. Kron (2010) interprets this as a "transnational turn" (121) taken by migration research in and about 'the Americas'. With this turn towards the transnational, cross-border migrants have come into focus as actors and subjects, and from a 'perspective from below' it was shown how by means of transnational (life) practices social arrangements may be shaped and, as a result, how power relationships can be avoided and confounded. In the perspective of transmigration, the shaping of life is taking place more or less simultaneously at various geographical locations. Therefore, the social practices of transmigrants in performing their lives stretch across several locations, as a result of which plurilocal social spaces, i.e., transnational spaces, emerge (cf. Pries 2000).

Precisely with respect to the migration between Mexico and the U.S, the reasons for assuming the burden of departure as well as the reasons for constantly returning are shown (cf. especially Pries 2000). The former, the reasons for leaving, lie above all in the hope of obtaining work, of finding better working conditions and a (higher) salary, as well as in the hope of fulfilling the 'American Dream'. The reasons for returning are above all family—and socially related, which come to bear more clearly in the case of migrated women.

At the same time, transnational spaces should not be seen as mere geographical locations but rather as "invisible structures of multiply networked government, legal and cultural transitions" (Apitzsch 2003: 69), since in transnational social spaces people develop plurilocal networks and organisations that cannot be understood in terms of the traditional 'nation-state-as-container model'. Instead, biographical experiences and biographies are constituted at the previously cited crossroads and transition points.

Ursula Apitzsch (2003) has identified biographical narratives as "locations on the map of transnational space" (69). Biography as the location of transnational and transcultural spaces is, according to Apitzsch, "an intersectional point of collective constitution and individual construction" (72). With this, Apitzsch is in keeping with the fundamental assumption of biographical research, which states that "the generally valid [lies] hidden in the concreteness of the individual case" (Alheit 1992: 20). Biographical research aims to reconstruct the traces of the socially general in individual biographies, since the methodological assumption of biographical research is that at the basis of the narratives there are generative structures of "a commonly shared reality" (Rosenthal and Fischer-Rosenthal 2003: 457), which can be brought to life and scientifically reconstructed in the interaction between researchers and narrators. At the same time, a dialectics of the individual and the social is assumed, one which is taken into account in the biographical analysis. And via the reconstruction of the biographical relationships in the context of migration, "insight can be gained into the process structures of legal, moral and emotional transgressions" (Apitzsch 2003: 71).

Characterising biography as a *location* and hence projecting a geographical terminology on to the social has been criticised by various authors. Helma Lutz (2004), for example, warns that by doing so the time reference that is created in very different ways in biographical narratives is missing. Following the views of Stuart Hall (2004), Lutz argues that biography cannot be conceived of as a location but rather as an *articulation* in which self-localisation and the localisation of others are being expressed, as well as the connections between them and the new connections between elements.

The stimulus on biographical research that proceeds from Hall's reflections is not exhausted, however, simply with reference to the issue of articulation. Rather, through Hall's concept of identity the basic methodological concepts (of society and subject) have to be revised. Quite in opposition to the notion of a free eligibility or a post-modern delimitation, Hall defines 'identities' as nodal points at which powerful subjectivating discourses and practices involving the situating of others coincide with discourse and practices of self-situation.

I use identity in order to refer to the *suture* point between discourses and practices on the one hand—the appeal to us to locate ourselves discursively as a particular social being—and processes that produce subjectivities on the other—which construct us as subjects who allow themselves to 'speak', who are comprehensible. Identities represent such points of temporary connections with subject positions that emerge from discursive practices. (Hall 2004: 173)

In Hall's view, identities are "positions that the subject *must* take"; they are, therefore, "not a being but a *positioning*" (173).[5] At the methodological level, therefore, social researchers are confronted with the task of bringing together the powerful and regulating discourses and the constitution of the subject (cf. Tuider 2007). In using a combination of biographical research and discourse analysis, the simultaneity of different, overlapping subjective experiences and discursive attributions that are characteristic of transnational biographies can be understood.

## TRANSNATIONAL FAMILIES

The increasing internationalisation and transnationalisation of migration movements also affect the shaping of family and parental relationships:

The transnational fields undoubtedly create varying impacts, such as, for example, on the shaping of identities and the feeling of belonging, on family and gender relationships, economic relations, processes of social mobility, religious practices, the labour market, perceptions and images of migration and on political participation, among others. (Parella 2008: 2)

Affected through migration the family now no longer refers to a common place of residence, but rather family relationships may extend over various geographically scattered locations. In current migration research the term 'transnational families' has recently been used.[6] According to Bryceson and Vuorela (2002), the transnational family may be defined as a family

whose members live some or most of the time apart, and who are able to create ties that give family members the feeling that they are part of the unit and that their welfare is attended to within a collective dimension, in spite of the physical distance. (2)[7]

In this context we have to abandon notions of 'family' as a natural, biological unit. Instead, the family must be understood[8] as a socially constructed community, in which case the creation and maintenance of family boundaries are a task of construction that has to be actively performed by all family members. Because the family is actively created at the everyday level, we can, following on the notion of 'doing gender' and 'doing ethnicity' speak also of 'doing family'. "Family processes and relationships among persons defined as relatives comprise the basic foundation for all other transnational social relations." (Basch et al. 1994: 238)

Whereas Suárez (2007) brings out the fact the transnational family does not represent a new phenomenon, Parella (2008) stresses that new possibilities for shaping the family may emerge today, since new technological advances mean that social family relationships may not only be maintained across vast distances and periods of time, but may also be nurtured through frequent and regular communication, for example, via Skype and webcams. In practical terms this means that, for example, the ritual Saturday evening meal may be practiced in front of the computer, household decisions may be made in common, and discussions involving the raising of children may be carried on together, regardless of the different geographic locations and different time zones the individual family members reside in (Tagmano 2003).

Therefore, communication technologies, such as the (mobile) telephone and the Internet (including webcams), become an important resource and enrichment for present transnational families in their efforts to live out and shape emotional commitment and responsibility, concern for other family members and involvement in family matters.[9] In this context, different gender configurations may now arise (cf. Solé, Parella, and Cavalcanti 2007): the migration of the father and husband corresponds to the traditional gender attribution of the male as breadwinner and caretaker. At the same time, the male migration may be associated with a release of the woman who stays behind from traditional duties and functions, since it is now this woman left behind who administers the *remesas* (remittances).[10] This may go hand in hand with the woman's greater independence and self-affirmation. In the case of sexualised violence in the family, the migration of the men is felt to be a form of escape and salvation (Solé et al. 2007). If the wife (and mother) initiates the migration process and thus becomes the breadwinner, this may trigger for her a process of empowerment, and also bring into question the traditional role of the husband. As Parella (2008) has stated, "The hegemonic patriarchal model is thrown into crisis" (10). Regardless of who leaves, migration represents a turning point in family and gender configurations as intrafamily power balance is affected. But who takes care of the children who are often left behind in the region of origin?

## TRANSNATIONAL MOTHERHOOD

The western notion of 'motherhood' includes the belief that physical and psychological closeness, that physical presence and emotional participation are coupled with one another and intertwined. The one conditions the other, or the two are inconceivable without each other. Transnational mothers muddle this notion. In her studies on Latin American women migrants in Los Angeles whose children remain in their country of origin, Hondagneu-Sotelo (2001) has been one of the first to show how new variations on the organisational arrangements of motherhood emerge, since in order to bridge the gap between spatial and chronological distance, migrated women create alternative childraising models. A transformation of the previous form of motherhood goes hand in hand with this.

In her studies of female Filipino migrants, Parreñas (2001) points to the fact that new forms and notions of motherhood arise after years of separation among family members, to the extent that motherhood is no longer linked to physical proximity to one's children. Motherhood is, instead, experienced through financial support or the financing of a child's education. Lauser (2005), too, in her analyses of the 'transnational mother' conditioned by marriage migration, points out the articulation of motherly love through gifts, financial remittances, or paying for a good school education. Therefore, some have asked the critical question of whether mothers are becoming 'gift mothers' (*madres de los regalos*) as a result of the migration process (Pedone 2006).[11] Thus, transnational motherhood for migrating women usually also implies an unsolvable, ideologically charged contradiction: on the one hand, being a 'good mother' entails earning money for one's children and family; on the other hand, a 'good mother' is expected to be together with her children—and not physically separated from them (Hondagneu-Sotelo and Avila 1997; Wagner 2005).

Migration processes involving women are often easier, or even possible in the first place, in a setting of extended family relationships and networks, the *redes de cuidado* (networks of care). In such settings especially the grandmothers help out with taking care of the children (Wagner 2005; Oral 2006; Nobles 2006; Parella 2007), but also other relatives, neighbours, or girlfriends could look after the children and the household of the migrated woman.[12] By doing so, the reproductive work is usually passed on from one female hand (that of the mother) to another (that of the grandmother, sister, aunt, girlfriend, etc.) (Nobles 2006). Both the women who migrate and those who stay behind remain captive to a particular logic of reproduction. Hochschild (2000) problematises with this "globalisation of motherhood" (130) the worldwide unequal distribution of both material and emotional resources.[13]

Hochschild speaks of an "emotional surplus value" which results from the fact that the countries of the so-called 'First World' import maternal love from countries of the so-called 'Third World.' What might be expected now in western terms is the disintegration of the female migrant's family. But rather than that, what ends up happening in this "exploitation of care" (Hochschild 2000: 133) is a shift in family and maternal responsibility.

## PORTRAIT: SONIA ORTIZ MARTÍNEZ[14]

Sonia Ortiz Martínez is thirty-eight years old (born in 1970) and the sixth of thirteen children. She was born in a small village near the city of Durango in the middle region of Mexico. Since both of her parents were employed in agriculture, she too spent her early childhood in the countryside. On entering school she—as well as her brothers and sisters—moved to Durango City and lived with a paternal uncle, visiting her parents and siblings on the weekend. Her parents followed a teacher's advice and decided to send her, as the only one of the thirteen children, to secondary school and thus give her access to an academic education. Shortly after completing her training as a paralegal, at the age of nineteen, she met her future husband Héctor. After being engaged for six months, they were married and currently have two children: Carina, who is eighteen, and Nora, who is five.

Nine years ago Sonia migrated with her daughter Carina for the first time to Ciudad Juárez, where her parents and three of her sisters were already living. About this, she says:

> *Well, we came here, the reason why we came here is because the family is here. My mum, my dad emigrated . . . I guess it was about 13 years ago? because of economic problems. Life here is better, um . . . well, more work. They came here. I stayed there, married, with one daughter.*

Ciudad Juárez offered above all for the female members of the Ortiz family the opportunity to work and thus the prospect of 'a better life.'[15] At the end of the 1980s, Sonia's eldest sister Andrea was the first in the family to migrate to Ciudad Juárez, and in 1994 Sonia's mother, Doña Rosa, and her five youngest siblings joined her. Barely arrived in the border region, all of them began to work in a *maquila*. For that purpose, some birth certificates had to be forged in order to obtain a residence permit. In her interview, Doña Rosa tells, giving the term a quite positive connotation, that with the help of gringos who recycled factory cardboxes and wooden pallets in their neighborhood the Rosas family was able to use these materials to build their first dwelling in Ciudad Juarez. Up to this day her house has no water supply or sewer connection, but over the years she and her daughters succeeded in buying a total of four plots of land in the immediate vicinity and building 'houses' on them.[17]

Sonia, too, migrated with her daughter because of the prospect of a better financial situation through work in a *maquila*. Like many other female labourers, Sonia too judges the employment in the *maquiladora* to be pleasant and satisfactory. It offers her—despite the fact that she is not employed in the occupation for which she was trained—a good income and various other advantages such as a regular meal during shift work. Sonia's brothers and sisters and her mother agree that the *maquila* work has improved living conditions for her and her children. Even though they have to move from one *maquila* to the next, they stress the benefits of this type of work. In quite concrete terms, Sonia and her sisters speak of the fact that they now earn more money, or earn anything at all, they speak of the regular meals which they receive in the *maquila,* and of the possibility of buying clothes at the weekly second-hand street sales. In one interview passage Sonia compares her previous work in Durango with the *maquiladora* work in Ciudad Juárez:

> *That is, none of the advantages they give you here in the maquila [in Ciudad Juárez] are given to you there [in Durango]. Then . . . I had to take on two jobs in order to manage. I worked from Monday to Monday, every day of the week. And so, in the end I noticed that by doing so I was earning the same as here. Here I work from Monday to Friday. That gives me time off three days and I earn what I earned there in a week. And, but I have savings, I have a car, special shifts, two meals, all things that were missing there. Then, so, no, money makes you freer, a little freer than there. And so, that was the reason why we came here.*

This thoroughly positive assessment of *maquila* work, which is characterised in international solidarity literature as 'exploitative' and 'sexist',[18] was surprising for the interviewers. Sonia refers to these depictions and at the same time she rejects them: "There are no unions here but with all of the advantages that you have here, they are wealth." At the foreground of Sonia's biographical presentation there is instead the acquisition of options for acting and shaping which she gains from her *maquila*-work in the border region, since Sonia's migration to Ciudad Juárez and her work in the *maquila* was also an escape from her marriage. Sonia repeatedly separated from her husband because of his violent behaviour and his drug abuse, but she also kept returning to him. Under pressure from her husband, she again became pregnant six years ago and had her second daughter Nora. One year before the time of the interview she definitively broke ties with her husband and with the aid of her mother again migrated to Ciudad Juárez. Her youngest daughter Nora accompanied her. Since then both of them live on the sofa bed in Sonia's sister's and her family's living room–kitchen. This living arrangement and life situation entails a great deal of solidarity among family members. The costs and duties, such as for the care and supervision of the children, can in this way be reduced. At the same time, however, the space for solitude and privacy is restricted.

## MOTHERHOOD AT A DISTANCE

Carina, Sonia's oldest daughter, remained in Durango, at first with a maternal aunt and then with a paternal uncle. Today she lives in the house of Sonia's best girlfriend and the latter's daughter and attends, with the help of financing from a scholarship, upper school and plans to study medicine. Sonia has repeatedly tried to bring her oldest daughter to Ciudad Juárez but without success. Carina prefers to live in Durango.

Last year Sonia saw her daughter three times. Christmas, Easter, and Carina's birthday were the occasions on which she undertook the twenty-two-hour bus ride to Durango. Despite this limited physical presence, Sonia continues to maintain an emotional, involved, and active motherhood in relation to her oldest daughter by means of regular telephone calls and through mobile phone messages. The practices of motherhood at a distance are described by Sonia in her biographical self-presentation as follows:

> *Um, everyday she sends me messages or I send her a message. Um, so, I talk to her on the phone on Mondays. Then for sure. Sometimes on Wednesdays. And so, if I still have enough money left, then also on Friday. And if there is not much money left, I send her a message [SMS], almost always. Now I've found a possibility. . . . A co-worker of mine has, um, an Internet connection.*

Thus, the new media help Sonia to organise the 'motherhood at a distance' (Parreñas 2005). Today, through electronic means family networks can be nurtured over vast distances, even overcoming national borders (Solé and Parella 2005). In this sense the Internet and the mobile phone are supporting migration movements, crossing and transforming borders and social spaces and enabling family relationships.[19] Sonia can remain an emotional reference person for her daughter Carina and fulfill her childraising duties in spite of the distance.

In doing so, Sonia has to master various challenges: First, she and her daughter need to gain access to the Internet; second, she has to coordinate her working hours with the rhythm of her daughter's life. In the latter case, Sonia's position as a person in charge in the *maquila* gives her certain room for manoeuvre:

> *A colleague has, um, an Internet connection. Well, so, now we are in contact with each other via Internet. In my girlfriend's workshop, across the way, there is an Internet café. Then, somehow, we'll manage to communicate soon. On Monday, on Monday I am more . . . , the fact is that I don't have a lot of opportunities, since during work you can't leave your workstation. Then, um, this, my colleague, he told me: 'If you'd like to speak to your child,' well, um, 'then we can get on the Internet and you can talk to her for 20 minutes.' But at that time of day it is already pretty late there. We'll try and find another time to speak.*

Sonia thus manages to maintain a regular contact with her oldest daughter by using a mobile phone and the Internet. In doing so, she is not only a financier for her daughter, but also takes an active part in her daughter's life. Decisions, for example, about her later educational career, are discussed together just as are the everyday events in Durango. Sonia and Carina are successful in being present reciprocally in each other's lives and in maintaining an emotional and caring mother-daughter relationship. In the following interview passage it becomes clear how Sonia takes part in her daughter's life and how she shows emotions as well as authority in her relationship with Carina.

> *Sure, if something goes wrong, my girlfriend sends me a message. 'This happened and that, that, that.' Um, 'don't tell her I told you that'. ((laughs)) And then I am already calling up there: 'Hey, tell me, what's happened? Do you have something to tell me?'—'Hm, something has happened. You already know that, why ( . . . ) are you asking me!' ((laughs))—'Well, because I want you to tell me about it.' Or sometimes she herself calls me up. Or I call her and she says 'This and that happened and my aunt became angry.' Well. And, then, I scold her. And she knows that when I'm peeved, I'm peeved. And apart from the fact that it bothers me, I don't speak to her anymore. And that hurts her more than anything else. It hurts her that I don't even speak to her.*

Through this regular contact and the actively shaped relationship, the 'emotional costs' of migration, which were often the result of information and communication gaps and significant time delays (via snail mail) are also reduced.

## CONCLUSION

In her migration Sonia has crossed no national border. She 'only' lives at the northern border to the U.S. and not in the U.S. itself. Nonetheless, in the way in which her motherhood is shaped with regard to her oldest daughter Carina, characteristic features can be seen of transnational aspects and practices which are currently being discussed under the term 'transnational motherhood.' Sonia's biography can be seen as a prime example which illustrates the delimitation of the life world ascertained at the outset. This delimitation, according to the subsequent thesis, includes not only transnational biographies in the framework of migration but is also at work beyond the limits of migration research.

## NOTES

1. Parnreiter (1999) has pointed out that the various programmes of the U.S. government as well as its tightening-up and militarisation of the southern U.S. border cannot contribute to a reduction in the migration flows from the south, but rather only to an official distinction being made between legal and

illegal residents. The function of the border then lies in separation and in the 'regulation of the population' as well as in the (dis)qualification and illegalisation of workers (on this point, see also Massey 1998). "In this sense transnational spaces could be understood as a precarious cultural expression of a politico-economic strategy that relies on the transnationalization of part of the population, i.e., on mobility plus the outsourcing of social reproduction. The phenomenon of transnational parenthood, which means above-average rates of transnational motherhood, is the very symbol par excellence of this migration regime. Here the creative utilisation of transnational space as one of the few resources available to female migrants from the east and the south is closely entangled with the politico-economic strategy of the appropriation of just such lived transnational flexibility" (Hess 2004: 4).

2. The here presented discussion is based on biographical interviews that were conducted by Marcela Gualotuña, Mauricio Carrera, and Elisabeth Tuider during a study trip in March 2008 in Ciudad Juárez. A total of five biographical interviews in a family context were compiled, i.e., a sixty-four-year-old woman and her four daughters who had migrated each participated in separate interviews. This chapter concentrates mostly on the interview with Sonia Ortiz Martínez. All names have been changed to protect people's anonymity.

3. Within this chapter I do not go into discussions of the working conditions in the *maquila* and the question of the impact of *maquila* work on the empowerment of women (on this point, cf. De la O 2007; Quintero 2007).

4. On the discussion and the model of transnational social spaces in the German context, cf. especially Pries (1997), Faist (2000); decisive for the U.S.-American debates on the topic are: Massey et al. (1994), Goldring (1996), Smith (1995), and Glick Schiller et al. (1992).

5. At this point Hall objects to both the feminist and antiracist politics of identity of the 1970s, as well as to the deconstructionist dissolution of the acting subject. Instead, he speaks in favour of the opportunity and the necessity of 'politics of positioning'.

6. The 'transnational family' is not a unified type but rather subsumes different forms of geographical and physical separation of family members (for a discussion of the term, cf. Guarnizo 1997). The strategies and practices of transnational families differ depending on the particular economic and political setting, as well as according to the individual class, age, and gender affiliation and the ethnic, national, and sociocultural background (Solé et al. 2007).

7. But not every family whose members reside in different regions or nation-states is necessarily a transnational family. Rather, social relationships and practices constitute the main criteria for defining a family as such.

8. The family represents a co-habiting association of people (one which in Germany is quite privileged), which comprises at least two interrelated generations and includes motherhood and/or fatherhood. Since up to now no studies exist on transmigration in homosexual or transgendered families or homosexual partnerships with children, in the following discussion the term 'family' will refer to the heteronormative family.

9. In this way, the increasing diffusion and penetration of telecommunications does not necessarily have this effect but instead, it favours and supports processes of transnationalisation, for only through telecommunications may daily and continuous contacts be maintained in a financially affordable way despite geographical distances. Especially among people from the lower social classes and in regions that are not connected to the telephone network, the spread of mobile phones strengthens the maintenance and cultivation of social relations, since they offer a comparatively inexpensive form of communication across distance (Galperín and Mariscal 2007).

10. Remittances (*remesas*) to those back home represent the most important source of income in Mexico. Currently, the *remesas* amount to approximately 20–24 billion U.S. dollars and exceed the income derived from the petroleum industry or tourism. For many families the *remesas* are a principal source of income that serves to stabilise the family income. An increasing number of families, most of them from the rural regions of Mexico (40 percent of all households with a migration background) are dependent on *remesas* for securing their livelihood. Therefore, the *remesas* are rarely used to finance investments. (cf. Hamann 2005).

11. Pedone (2006) writes, concerning Ecuadoran children who grow up with their grandparents because their parents have migrated, of a story according to which a grandmother who had been having difficulties with a child asked the child's mother to refrain from sending 'gifts' as long as the child misbehaved. As a result of not receiving gifts from his mother, the child changed his behaviour.

12. At the same time, migrating women are often subjected to significant stigmatisation as 'uncaring mothers', 'family destroyers', or 'sexual libertines' (cf. Herrera and Martínez 2002).

13. "Are First World countries such as the United States importing maternal love as they have imported copper, zinc, gold and other ores from Third World countries in the past?" (Hochschild 2000: 135).

14. The interview with Sonia Ortiz Martínez was conducted on 16 March 2008 in Ciudad Juárez. All the textual quotes not otherwise referenced in the remainder of this chapter derive from the script of this interview.

15. The *maquiladoras*, the free export production zones along the northern Mexican border—just as in Latin America as a whole—gained in economic and political importance in the last twenty years. They are the main goal of domestic migration in Mexico and have attracted and are attracting particularly women (Berndt 2004; Zamorano Villareal 2004). For the year 2006, INEGI records that 388,019 female labourers and 340,446 male labourers worked in the *maquilas* in the border region near the U.S. (INEGI 2007a: 13).

16. The term *gringos* is used in Mexico to describe 'white' U.S. Americans. The phrase 'with the help of gringos' used in the interview also includes the international and transnational corporations that have settled in Ciudad Juárez. The terminology used thus forms part of the very positive attitude of the women interviewed towards the *maquiladora* and the corporations.

17. Having one's own piece of land in Ciudad Juárez means having a piece of independence, in light of the horrendous rental prices. Property is also a symbol of successful migration. The importance of the family at whose centre Doña Rosa stands is thus reflected in the explicitly desired vicinity of her sisters and her mother. At the same time, the family association is extended by having separate houses for one's own children and grandchildren.

18. See, for example, the Maquila Solidarity Network (MSN): http://en.maquilasolidarity.org/.

19. In Mexico there are approximately nineteen landline and fifty-five mobile phone connections per one hundred inhabitants (INEGI 2007b). That means that three out of every four people have access to a telephone.

## BIBLIOGRAPHY

Alheit, P. (1992) 'Biographizität und Struktur.' In *Biographische Konstruktionen. Beiträge zur Biographieforschung*, edited by P. Alheit, B. Dausien, Hanses, A. and A. Scheuermann, 10–36, Bremen: Universität Bremen.

Apitzsch, U. (2003) 'Migrationsbiographien als Orte transnationaler Räume.' In *Migration, Biographie und Geschlechterverhältnisse*, edited by U. Apitzsch and M. M. Jansen, 65–80. Münster: Westfälisches Dampfboot.

Apitzsch, U., and I. Siouti (2008) 'Transnationale Biographien.' In *Soziale Arbeit und Transnationalität*, edited by H. G. Homfeldt, W. Schröer, and C. Schweppe, 97–111. Weinheim and München: Juventa.

Appadurai, A. (1991) 'Global Ethnoscapes: Notes and Queries for a Transnational Anthropology.' In *Recapturing Anthropology: Working in the Present*, edited by R. G. Fox, 191–210. Santa Fe: School of American Research Press.

Basch, L., N. Glick Schiller, and C. Blanc-Szanton (1994) *Nations Unbound: Transnational Projects, Postcolonial Predicaments and Deterritorialized Nation-States*. New York: Routledge.

Beck, U. (1997) *Was ist Globalisierung?* Frankfurt/Main: Suhrkamp.

Berndt, C. (2004) *Globalisierungs-Grenzen. Modernisierungsträume und Lebenswirklichkeiten in Nordmexiko*. Bielefeld: Transkript.

Bryceson, D., and U. Vuorela, eds. (2002) *The Transnational Family: New European Frontiers and Global Networks*. Oxford: Berg Publications.

De la O, M. E. (2007) 'El trabajo de las mujeres en la industria Maquiladora de México: balance de cuatro décadas de estudio.' *Debate Feminista*, 18(35), México: 31–56.

Faist, T. (2000) *The Volume and Dynamics of International Migration and Transnational Social Spaces*. Oxford: Oxford University Press.

Faist, T. (2007) 'Transnationale Migration als relative Immobilität in einer globalisierten Welt.' *Berliner Journal für Soziologie*, 17, Berlin: 365–85.

Galperin, H., Mariscal J. (2007) 'Oportunidades Móviles: Pobreza y Telefonía Móvil en América Latina y el Caribe.' http://dirsi.net/node/106. Retrieved 27 October 2011.

Glick Schiller, N., L. Basch, and C. Blanc-Szanton (1992) 'Towards a Definition of Transnationalism: Introductory Remarks and Research Questions.' In *Towards a Transnational Perspective on Migration: Race, Class, Ethnicity and Nationalism Reconsidered*, edited by N. Glick Schiller, L. Basch, and C. Blanc-Szanton, ix–xiv, New York: Johns Hopkins University Press.

Goldring, L. (1996) 'Blurring Borders: Constructing Transnational Communities in the Process of Mexico-US Immigration.' *Research in Community Sociology*, 6: 69–104.

Guarnizo, L. E. (1997) 'The Emergence of a Transnational Social Formation and the Mirage of Return Migration among Dominican Transmigrants.' *Identities*, 4: 281–322.

Hall, S. (1994) *Rassismus und kulturelle Identität. Ausgewählte Schriften 2*. Hamburg: Argument.

Hamann, V. (2005) 'Migration und wirtschaftliche Entwicklung: Die Investitionen der MigrantInnen aus Zacatecas, Mexiko.' *Peripherie*, 97/98 (2005): 88–106.

Herrera, G., and A. Martínez (2002) *Género y Migración en la Región Sur*. Quito: Flacso.

Hess, S. (2004) 'Transnationale Räume. Widerständige soziale Sphären und neuer Modus transnationalen Regierens.' http://www.copyriot.com/diskus/03_04/03_trans.html. Retrieved 9 July 2008.

Hochschild, A. R. (2000) 'Global Care Chains and Emotional Surplus Value.' In *On the Edge: Living with Global Capitalism*, edited by W. Hutton and A. Giddens, 130–46. London: Jonathan Cape.

Hondagneu-Sotelo, P. (2001): Domestica. Derkeley/CA: University of California Press.

Hondagneu-Sotelo, P., and Avila, E. (1997) "I'm Here, But I'm There': The Meanings of Latina Transnational Motherhood.' *Gender and Society*, II(5): 548–71.

Kron, S. (2010) 'Grenzen im Transit. Zur Konstitution politischer Subjektivitäten in transmigrantischen Räumen.' In *Prokla 138, Postkoloniale Studien als kritische Sozialwissenschaft*, 121–37. Münster: Westf. Dampfboot.

Lauser, A. (2005) 'Philippinische Frauen unterwegs. Eine transnationale Perspektive auf Heiratsmigration.' *Südostasien*, 2005(3): 70–74.

Lutz, H. (2004) 'Transnationale Biographien in globalisierten Gesellschaften.' In *Migration in der metropolitanen Gesellschaft*, edited by M. Ottersbach and E. Yildiz, 207–16. Münster: Lit.

Massey, D. Goldring, L, & Durand, J. (1994). 'Continuities in Transnational Migration: An Analysis of 19 Mexican Communities.' *American Journal of Sociology*, 99, 1492–1533.

Massey, D. (1998) 'March of Folly: US Immigration Policy after NAFTA.' *The American Prospect*, 137: 22–33.

Nobles, J. (2006) 'The Contribution of Migration to Children's Family Contexts.' http://escholarship.org/uc/item/5zk5t0d1. Retrieved 27 October 2011.

Oral, K. (2006) 'Somos todo aquí y allá: Trabajo reproductivo y productivo de mujeres en una comunidad transnacional en Chiguagua, México.' http://redalyc.uaemex.mx/src/inicio/ArtPdfRed.jsp?iCve=88402415. Retrieved 27 October 2011.

Parella, S. (2007) 'Los vínculos afectivos y de cuidado en las familias transnacionales, Migrantes ecuatorianos y peruanos.' Migraciones Internacionales 2(4): 151–188. http://redalyc.uaemex.mx/src/inicio/ArtPdfRed.jsp?iCve=15140206. Retrieved 27 October 2011.

Parella, S. (2008) 'An Approach to the Transnational Practices of Latina Migrants in Spain and Its Impact on Transnational Homes.' Paper given at the 1st ISA Forum of Sociology, Barcelona, 5–8 September 2008.

Parnreiter, C. (1999) 'Acht Thesen zur Migration zwischen Mexiko und USA.' *Widerspruch. Flüchtlinge, Migration und Integration.* 37: 51–59.

Parreñas, R. S. (2001) 'Mothering from a Distance: Emotions, Gender and Intergenerational Relations in Filipino Transnational Families.' *Feministische Studien*, 27: 361–89.

Parreñas, R. S. (2005) *Children of Global Migration: Transnational Families and Gendered Woes.* Stanford: Stanford University Press.

Pedone, C. (2006) 'Los cambios familiares y educativos en los actuales contextos migratorios ecuatorianos: una experiencia transatlántica.' Athenea Digital. Revista de pensamiento e investigación social, 10: 154–171. http://redalyc.uaemex.mx/pdf/537/53701010.pdf. Retrieved 27 October 2011.

Pries, L. (1997) 'Wege und Visionen der Erwerbsarbeit. Erwerbsverläufe und biographische Projekte abhängiger und selbständig Beschäftigter in Mexiko.' *Zeitschrift für Wirtschaftsgeographie*, 48 (2): 139–140.

Pries, L. (2000) 'Transnationalisierung der Migrationsforschung und Entnationalisierung der Migrationspolitik. Das Entstehen transnationaler Sozialräume durch Arbeitswanderung am Beispiel Mexiko—USA.' In Bommes, Michael (pub.): Transnationalismus und Kulturvergleich. Osnabrück: IMIS, 55–79.

Quintero Ramírez, C. (2007) 'Trabajo femenino en las Maquiladoras: ¿explotación o liberación?' In *Bordeando las violencia contra las mujeres en la frontera norte de México*, edited by J. Monarrez Fragoso and M. Tabuenca Córdoba, Tijuana: El Colegio de la Frontera Norte.

Rosenthal, G. and Fischer- Rosenthal, W. (1997): Warum Biographieforschung und wie man sie macht. In: *ZSE*, 1007(4): 405–427.

Smith, R. (1995) 'Los ausentes siempre presentes: The Imagining, Making and Politics of Transnational Communities between Ticuani, Puebla, Mexico and New York City.' PhD diss., Columbia University.

Solé, C. and S. Parella (2005) ´Discursos sobre la "maternidad transnacional" de las mujeres de origen latinoamericano residentes en Barcelona.´ Mobilités au féminin-Tanger, 14: 12–24. http://lames.mmsh.univ-aix.fr/Papers/ParellaSole_ES.pdf. Retrieved 27 October 2011.

Solé, C., S. Parella, and L. Cavalcanti (2007) *Los vínculos económicos y familiares transnacionales: Los migrantes ecuatorianos y peruanos en España*. Madrid: Fundación BBVA.

Suárez, L. (2007) 'La perspectiva transnational en los estudios migratorios: Génesis, derroteros y surcos metodológicos.' Paper given at the 5th Congress on Immigration in Spain: "Migrations and Human Development," Valencia, March 2007.

Tagmano, C. (2003) "Entre Celulinos y Cholulares': los procesos de conectividad y la construcción de las identidades trasnacionales.' http://lasa.international.pitt.edu/Lasa2003/TamagnoCarla.pdf. Retrieved 22 July 2008.

Tuider, E. (2007) 'Diskursanalyse und Biographieforschung. Zum Wie und Warum von Subjektpositionierungen.' *Forum Qualitative Sozialforschung / Forum: Qualitative Social Research*, 8(2), http://www.qualitative-research.net/fqs-texte/2-07/07-2-6-d.htm. Retrieved 27 Oct 2011.

Wagner, H. (2005) 'Maternidad transnacional, discursos, teorías y prácticas.' http://homepage.univie.ac.at/heike.wagner/matertransn.pdf. Retrieved 11 July 2008.

Zamorano Villareal, C. (2004) 'Ser inmigrante en Ciudad Juárez, Itinerarios en tiempos de la maquila.' *Frontera Norte, Colegio de la Frontera Norte*, 18 (35): 29–53. http://redalyc.uaemex.mx/src/inicio/ArtPdfRed.jsp?iCve=13603502. Retrieved 27 October 2011.

## INTERNET SOURCES

INEGI (2000) 'Mexicanos, residentes mujeres, 1970/1990/2000 Estados Unidos de América.' http://www.inegi.gob.mx/est/contenidos/espanol/rutinas/ept.asp?t=mpob65&s=est&c=5565. Retrieved 12 August 2008.

INEGI (2007a) 'Maquiladora de Exportación, Febrero de 2007.' http://www.inegi.gob.mx/prod_serv/contenidos/espanol/bvinegi/productos/continuas/economicas/maquiladora/ime/ime.pdf. Retrieved 10 July 2008.

INEGI (2007b) 'Indicadores de los servicios telefónicos 2005 y 2006.' http://www2.inegi.gob.mx:1212/inegi/contenidos/espanol/avantgo/mexicoc/11t2.asp?prproyec=2&tema=11&subtema=2. Retrieved 1 November 2008.

Part V

# Transnational Social Support

Unintended Consequences and Future
Challenges

# 10  The Missing Presence of Aboriginal Peoples from the Transnational Debate

*Adrienne Chambon and Arielle Dylan*

## INTRODUCTION

This chapter stems from the startling observation of the missing presence of Aboriginal peoples from discussions and scholarship on transnationalism. As the investigations and conceptualisations of transnational relations have expanded to include families, communities, social movements, religion, economics, policy, and gendered and racialised relations, a vast array of relationships has been re-examined through a transnational lens, thus bringing in a new level of complexity. Yet, Aboriginal peoples have remained outside of that framework, perceived as the earliest inhabitants of the lands, whose worlds were transformed by the advent of foreign migration. The more recent thinking on transnationalism has evolved from studies of migration, taking into account the reconsidered status of nation-states and historicising their multiple effects. It is the settler peoples and the peoples who migrated after the constitution of nation-states who are considered in their transnational experiences. Yet, the absence of Aboriginal peoples from transnational thinking raises many questions. Leaving out Aboriginal peoples from this discussion can obfuscate a number of relations that Indigenous people enter into which are of a transnational nature. This absence restricts our understanding of transnational realities, and the existing and needed mechanisms of social support that are called for to sustain transnational relations. In this chapter we explore some of the possible sets of relationships that concern Aboriginal peoples in relation to transnationalism.

We first set out some of the possible reasons for this absence, which stem in part from dominant perspectives that confine Aboriginal relations to a certain terrain. Other reasons stem from the agendas that Aboriginal peoples themselves have actively pursued in making claims for redress. We then follow with the presentation of three instances of transnational relations entered into by Aboriginal peoples, two from within the territory that is known as Canada and a third with Aboriginal peoples in Canada as members of a broader alliance. We argue that in order for the transnational realities of Aboriginal peoples to be envisaged, revisiting a whole set of assumptions is required. We believe this opens up the way for a number of investigations.

## SOME CONTEXTUAL BACKGROUND

In the past few decades, transnationalism literature has proliferated across a variety of academic disciplines, including sociology, anthropology, migrant studies, history, geography, ethnic and racial studies, media and cultural studies, and, more recently, social work. The 'container theory' of nation-states, characteristic of social enquiry guided by 'methodological nationalism' (Levitt and Glick Schiller 2004; see chapter 1) has been challenged along with conventional immigration paradigms, as intensified global economic, social, and epistemic forces and flows have engendered and (re)constructed transnational practices, identities, spaces, and places (Vertovec 2004; 1999).

Broadly, transnationalism describes the various linkages connecting peoples, communities, and organisations across the delineated somewhat arbitrary boundaries of nation-states. Transnational practices are not new, nor are transnational communities. As Wolf argues, cultures and societies constituted well before the development of capitalism were influenced by elements of larger systems, and can only be understood when contextualised "in their mutual interrelationships and interdependencies in space and time" (Wolf [1982] 1997: x). "Once we locate the reality of society in historically changing, imperfectly bounded, multiple and branching social alignments [ . . . ] the concept of a fixed, unitary, and bounded culture must give way to a sense of the fluidity and permeability of cultural sets" (Wolf [1982] 1997: 387).

Although Wimmer and Glick Schiller (2003) justifiably emphasise the resiliency of the nation-state in the face of transnational processes, their insistence that globalisation and its defining technologies do not represent an 'epochal turn' is at odds with the premises of this chapter. Earlier historical periods were not static, culturally homogeneous, or politically and economically unsophisticated, but this does not discount the momentous social, societal, national, inter-, and transnational changes wrought by the technological infrastructure of globalisation. Paehlke (2004) asserts that "electronic (or 'digitalized' or 'globalized') capitalism can be understood as a socioeconomic mode different from all previous modes—as a third type of industrial society" (40). The increasing efficiency and scope of telecommunications technologies, and the availability and relative affordability of air travel have sufficiently compressed space and time, making it possible not only for accelerated flows of capital, goods, ideas, and images, but also for increasing numbers of individuals to possess a twofold experience of place, encompassing both here and there (Vertovec 2004; Hondagneu-Sotelo and Avila 1997). Sometimes a considerable difference in degree, such as the technological developments in the latter half of the twentieth century, can produce pronounced qualitative differences. As Landolt (2001) argues, contemporary "transnational migration [and, it could be added, transnational practices in general] . . . exhibits an expansion in the realms of what is possible, the scope of who can do it, and in the complexity and consequences of what is done" (220).

Exploring transnational processes while simultaneously holding onto the concept of the nation-state, however altered, necessitates new ways of thinking. We need to develop new and evolving questions that address the multiple and changing identity, border, and order formations and fluidities characterising transnational spaces (Vertovec 2004). Equally important are questions concerning which forms of transnational practices are foregrounded and which transnational groups, peoples, and collectivities are studied or ignored and why. There is a noticeable lack of literature on Indigenous transnational practices. Alia's (2010) writings on global networking through media and transcending national specificities to achieve unity, and de Costa's writings on Indigenous peoples' activism in transnational networks and in global institutions (2006) stand out among the few exceptions to this trend. The following section of this chapter begins by postulating why this gap might exist.

## GAP IN THE DISCOURSE—ABORIGINAL PEOPLES OUTSIDE AND INSIDE THE NATION-STATE

The questions of transnationalism rest upon the displacement of the nation-state as the dominant reference, container, and shaper of sets of social relationships, policies, and institutional practices. As an approach, transnationalism aims to militate against and become disembedded from the hegemonic dominance of the nation-state. National entrenchment is a problem of perspective. In the Canadian context, the vexed relationship First Peoples have with Canada's federal polity illustrates this point. The ways in which Aboriginal peoples think about, and the ways in which they are thought of in relation to, the nation-state raise critical questions.

Aboriginal peoples inhabited the land now known as Canada long before the arrival of western Europeans or the creation of the nation-state. In the early contact period, non-Aboriginals sought the assistance of Aboriginal peoples in the Atlantic and the St. Lawrence River region in order to survive the relatively harsh, unfamiliar lands. In time, as non-Aboriginals gained not only numerical supremacy but also a greater colonial foothold, Aboriginal peoples were relegated to the periphery, increasingly forced to reserves and subjected to assimilationist policies (Miller 2000). The Aboriginal-state relationship was a product of colonialism, pre-capitalism, and early capitalism (Sayre 2008). The conflictual relations between Aboriginals and newcomers became most pronounced with the advent of the market and the political system of 'democracy.'

However, Aboriginal peoples' presence is being felt powerfully in contemporary Canadian society through effective political organising and profound displays of resistance, such as changing legislation recognising Aboriginal title rights to the land that had not been extinguished under English law. These rights can be asserted today and have served as the basis for negotiations and land claims settlements such as the *Calder (1973)*[1] and *Delgamuukw (1997)*[2] court decisions in British Columbia, documented in the proceedings (Persky 1998; Christie 2005). Such decisions signify considerable advancement in understanding Aboriginal and Treaty rights in the Canadian legal system, and reflect the rise in resource-based economic developments on Treaty lands.[3] Although the British colonising power failed to involve Aboriginal peoples in the establishment of the nation-state, imposing upon them instead a separate political status, the modalities of this recognition of difference removed them from the national compact. Today, the changing view is that it must be acknowledged that Aboriginal peoples' "contributions in economic terms alone were substantial [to the founding of this country] and can never be properly assessed. . . . In the most profound sense of the term, they are Canada's founding peoples" (Dickason 2002: xi).

Canada's early Constitution posits a special relationship as Dominion to England with Aboriginal peoples governed by the imperial power of Britain. Unmistakable examples of the reach of this power are the Indian Act,[4] the development of reserves, residential schools, and the withholding of the right to vote in the federal elections until 1960 (Cardinal 1999; Miller 2000). In contemporary democracy Aboriginal peoples are divided by different categories of statuses that were attributed historically by the Canadian government. In this social sense, they are not part of integrative considerations of the nation and, understandably, have a highly troublesome relationship with the rest of Canada. With Aboriginal rights being increasingly acknowledged by the Supreme Court of Canada and by the federal government, unsympathetic non-Aboriginals have been advocating a single set of rules for all Canadian citizens (Coates 2004). "According to polls conducted in 2003, a majority of Canadians now oppose the continued extension of indigenous and treaty rights" (Coates 2004).

Aboriginal peoples today consider that they are in nation-to-nation relationships with the federal government of Canada, seeing themselves as separate but parallel states (Royal Commission on Aboriginal Peoples 1996). Modern nation-states, as Eric Hobsbawm has demonstrated (1990), are based on industrial societies and anchored in a political government structure involving full participation of its citizens. Modern nation-states are differentiated from earlier notions of nations constituted as and defined by a people, in ethnic, language, or cultural terms. Therefore, because Aboriginal peoples are often cast as pre-industrial, their nations are sometimes conceived by members of the dominant society as lacking real nation status, being nothing more than quaint polities. This could explain, in part, why transboundary movements and transnational flows involving the circulation of persons, materials, and ideas across the borders of First Nations communities into the dominant society and into other First Nations and back again are not straightforwardly perceived as transnational practices.

Sadly, the lack of literature exploring Aboriginal transnational practices raises the spectre of three entwined conceptual and strategic blights characterising Canada's (and other colonising nations') colonial history. The first is the idea of *terra nullius*, a legal concept meaning 'empty land,' that was used to appropriate land from Aboriginal peoples by theorising their absence (Dickason 1993). Neglecting to consider Aboriginal peoples in discussions of transnational processes and spaces in Canada, and globally, risks theoretically reinscribing this pernicious concept. The second is the notion of atemporality, a belief that certain groups are "pristine survivals from a timeless past" (Wolf 1997: 385), making them candidates for primitivist ethnographic study and not sufficiently post-industrial to be considered as interlocutors in the communication and exchange activities that are addressed in transnational discourse. The last is the concept of being 'beyond the pale,' a phrase used historically to designate those persons and communities outside the bounds of civilised society (Dickason 1993). To be sure, Aboriginal peoples' current standard of living deviates in a substantive way from that of the statistical means of the general Canadian population in terms of death rate, suicide rate, health and poverty indices, housing, and education (Statistics Canada 2007), so in this social and political sense, they are located in an inferior position, at the periphery if not outside the frame of reference of the nation. The lack of texts investigating Aboriginal peoples' transnationalisms reinforces this periphery position suggesting Aboriginal practices are somehow separate from the realms in which transnational practices occur.

Of course evocation does not imply intent, and identifying the ways textual lacunae elicit this spectre does not actually explain the lack of literature exploring Aboriginal transnational practices; it does underscore the problematic historical resonances that such a gap produces. The small number of texts treating Indigenous transnationalism is probably best explained by three interrelated factors. First, few Aboriginal writers and scholars have directed their authorial attention to transnational concerns. While non-Aboriginal scholars have gamely embraced a shift toward global and transnational understandings including concepts of fluid borders and dismantling orders, Aboriginal scholars are busy asserting 'Aboriginal nationhood rights' which have been "banished from mainstream history and law and replaced by the theory of two founding nations: the English and the French" (Henderson 2000: 65). Invocations of 'deterritorialisation' and national instabilities are anathema to Aboriginal political strategising and cultural restoration, where the aim is to shore up First Nations. Second, many non-Aboriginal scholars remain unfamiliar with the historical reach and contemporary breadth of Aboriginal transnational practices. Third, the settler/transmigrant binarism found in much of the transnational literature does not provide a ready category for contemplating and discussing Aboriginal transnationalisms because of their unambiguous pre-'settler' status.

The remainder of this chapter endeavours to demonstrate the range of Aboriginal transnational processes that do take place through specific instances. The first, a historical case, dates back to the period before the constitution of the Canadian nation-state and involves a particular set of players.

## TRANSNATIONALISM AMONG THE WENDAT, ALGONQUIN, AND FRENCH PEOPLES

Some authors, engaged in transnational investigations and scholarship, have identified the weakness of focusing overwhelmingly on contemporary transnational processes (Vertovec 1999, 2004; Faulstich Orellana et al. 2001; Wimmer and Glick Schiller 2003; Tinsman and Shukla 2007). While the intensity of capitalist flows and labour migrations in the latter half of the twentieth century outstrips those from the earlier half and prior centuries, transnational forces were no less significant in former times and smaller regions or non-nation-states. Understanding such early transnational dynamics historicises globalisation and present-day transnationalisms, and helps better to frame questions of the nation-state, fluidity of borders, sovereign reach and authority, new subjectivities, bifocality, and bilocality (Tinsman and Shukla 2007). This section provides a brief look at transnational practices in an early contact setting involving Aboriginal peoples and French people in a period predating Canadian confederation by more than two hundred years, to illustrate linkages between the contemporary situation and the past, contextualising to some degree current Aboriginal transnational practices in Canada.

When the French came to the St. Lawrence region in the early seventeenth century to establish a colony and acquire resources, they learned of the Wendat peoples, a confederated group of First Nations who practiced farming in the interior, the region known today as Midland, Ontario. Intrigued by reports of horticultural peoples, land use involving tillage and crop production valued as eminently superior to non-horticultural hunter-gatherer practices, the French were keen to meet the Wendat for expansionist, mercantile, and proselytising purposes. Scouts, traders, and missionaries were sent to live among the Wendat, and their writings, along with those of Samuel de Champlain, who formed a military alliance with the Wendat and sojourned briefly among them, provide the fullest historical documentary accounts, however biased, of any Aboriginal-non-Aboriginal encounter in the Canadian context for this period. The historic record, though wanting for its complete absence of primary documents authored by Wendat actors (traders, leaders, warriors, and diplomats) and French traders and scouts, reveals a series of transnational and transregional crossings arising from engagement with material flows and market changes.

In the early seventeenth century some bands from First Nations comprising the Anishnabe Algonquin, for example, the Kinounchepirini and

Weskarini, among others, customarily wintered on the edge of Arendahronon Wendat communities exchanging French goods for Wendat cornmeal (Thwaites 1896–1901: 24: 269; Trigger 1994: 160). People from the Nipissing First Nation similarly spent the winter among the Attignawantan Wendat peoples. Before "reaching them, they catch as many fish as possible, which they dry. This is the ordinary money with which they buy their main stock of corn, although they come supplied with all other goods" (Thwaites 1896–1901: 21: 239). These seasonal transnational spaces that involved the receiving society and migrant communities surely produced new social formations and complex interconnections across and within First Nations borders. A consciousness of dual embeddedness would emerge during everyday lived experience in the winter months and throughout the remainder of the calendar year through resonances of the social, political, material, economic, and epistemic practices and changes. Evolving narratives would be produced and reproduced in this transnational constellation, this particular social geography.

Although groups of traders wintered at Quebec among the French in 1625 (Le Clercq 1691: 343) and then again in the 1640s, the Wendat in general were never keen to stay in French communities for extended periods. Trigger (1987) suggests that the 1625 winter stay of a Wendat party was driven by curiosity and a desire to cement relations with the French, while the sojourns in the 1640s can best be explained by military threat of the Haudenosaune and an increasing Wendat dependence on French goods. French interpreters, scouts, traders, and missionaries lived among the Wendat for long periods, and often on an ongoing basis. Because the journals kept by the missionaries are laden with the unfortunate stereotypes and offensive binary hierarchical dualisms that mark much of the colonial project worldwide (e.g., civilised/barbaric, Christian/heathen, human/subhuman), it is what is glimpsed indirectly of French traders and interpreters that best reveals transnational Wendat-French dynamics in Wendake, the territory of the Wendat.

The first European to travel to the interior was Etienne Brulé, who returned, according to Champlain, "dressed like an Indian" (Biggar 1922–36, 2: 188). Sagard, who lived among the Wendat from 1625 to 1626, describes French traders as rapidly adopting elements of Wendat dress, technologies, and cultural practices (Sagard 1866: 166, 611), but he also complains of the polluting moral influence the French exerted on the Wendat (Wrong 1939: 137). The Jesuits tried to stamp out the perceived immoral behaviour of French traders and interpreters among the Wendat in 1625, and in 1632 they redoubled these efforts by attempting to monitor more closely the activities of French men in Wendake, insisting on Christian marriages between French men and Wendat women rather than the marriage customs of the Wendat (Thwaites 1896–1901: 14: 15–17). It is in these Wendat-French transnational spaces, in which French traders and interpreters were living intermittently for extended periods among the

Wendat, where the conventional and transgressive commingled, and the construction of nascent identities and composite social and cultural formations emerged. It is regrettable that the tenuousness of the written traces and the missing voices of these more subaltern social actors limit us in our considerations of the instances and scope of mutual influences.

We now turn to collective forms of claims-making and organised resistance initiated by Indigenous peoples, and focus on the recent development of cross-border alliances among Indigenous peoples as a transnational strategy of advocacy.

## TRANSNATIONAL INDIGENOUS ALLIANCES AND ADVOCACY

As the historic record shows, First Nations peoples, like other peoples, actively entered into transnational arrangements not only to create or enhance material and epistemic circulations but also to form important, mutually beneficial alliances across borders. Historic precedents such as those described here lend depth to the understanding of contemporary political transnational strategies and activism practiced by Indigenous peoples around the world, strategies designed to resist persistent colonial forces and the more pernicious, neo-colonial aspects of globalisation and corporatisation. There are more than 370 million Indigenous peoples worldwide in ninety countries and the alliances forged across a number of Indigenous populations have assumed increasing international status.

The ostensible paradox inherent in the concept of Indigenous transnationalism has been observed by de Costa (2006) who identifies how localism, rootedness, and a place-based alignment, customarily associated with Indigeneity, appears initially inconsistent with a global orientation and related transnational practices. However, de Costa also quickly and rightly notes that the local is not sacrificed by Indigenous transnational processes but rather is buttressed, as borders of nation-states, and their sovereign reach, are continually exceeded through appeals to a "higher authority," powers existing outside the bounds of the colonising state (de Costa 2006). If the nation-state is conceived as a container of sorts having a geopolitical, ideological, and legislative perimeter which encloses a loosely common people sharing a broadly defined cultural identity and sociolinguistic commonalities (Vertovec 2004), then the situatedness of Indigenous peoples within this nation-state model invites transnational movement as a means to escape the periphery status created by centuries of colonisation and continued forms of oppression. Just as imperialist strivings, historically and to this day, operate by exceeding national boundaries to pursue worldly interests and alliances, Indigenous groups recognise the necessity of transnational strategies to meet shared local and global concerns, the need to go outside the restrictive and oppressive borders and social orders of the nation-states by which they were excluded and marginalised through constitutional and regulative processes affecting so many arenas of social life: educational, economic, political, and cultural.

Transnationalism, though not a new phenomenon, has certainly been augmented by intensified global trade, electronic communication, and resource availability making technological developments and swift forms of global travel possible. Said (1994) suggests the "pattern of dominions or possessions laid the groundwork for what is in effect now a fully global world" (6). In this fully global world there are extraordinary social, economic, and environmental disparities, and it is around these issues that Indigenous peoples have organised transnationally. Despite numerical inferiority, Indigenous peoples have advantageously employed the mobilising power of 'strategic essentialism' (Spivak 1990), forming strong pan-Indigenous alliances and leveraging tremendous moral power on the global stage through cogent human and land rights lobbying, activism, and discourse, collectively tackling shared challenges. Much of this has been facilitated by what Alia (2010) aptly terms the New Media Nation, a nation that is contingent upon technological innovations and lacks the seeming tangibility of the geopolitical nation-state, but is defined instead by a very real transnational, transcultural electronic space that defies state boundaries and surpasses geographical borders. One of the many benefits of this electronic nation is that it enjoys a wide audience of both Indigenous and non-Indigenous persons, as virtually anyone with Internet access can readily gain information regarding the multidimensionality of pan-Indigenous coalitions and their transnational courses and practices (Alia 2010). Although the dissemination and adoption of new technologies has raised concerns of detrimental cultural change and possible ethnocide among Indigenous and other marginalised groups (Mander 1991; Becker, Burwell, and Gilman 2002), Indigenous peoples have successfully used electronic communication for cultural and linguistic revival and to promote common social and political interests. Indeed, Lorde's (1984) argument notwithstanding, the so-called "master's tools" can be used to "dismantle the master's house," as Indigenous peoples are effectively using these technologies to critique, challenge, and subvert national orders.

The publication of George Manuel's *The Fourth World: An Indian Reality* in 1974 popularised the term Fourth World, first coined by Tanzanian High Commission first secretary, Mbuto Milando, as a descriptor for poor, marginalised groups not recognised as nations. The common history of attempted eradication and forced assimilation, paternalism, social and geographic ostracism, racism, and land expropriation created an alternate reality for Indigenous groups where they were either forcefully excluded from larger society (through reserve systems) and left to live beyond industrial borders (until the discovery of a desirable resource in lands formerly deemed valueless), or they themselves elected to distance themselves from the discrimination and foreign values of modern society, preferring instead the cultural and ethical logic of their own societal structures.

The economic and social inequities that have resulted from these rac-ist and systematic exclusionary practices are being increasingly contested in multinational forums through pan-Indigenous coalitions and commu-nications across national borders. On September 13, 2007, the United Nations Declaration on the Rights of Indigenous Peoples, involving iden-tity assertion, equity concerns, inclusivity, and structural transformation, was adopted by the General Assembly. Contained in this declaration is an article specifically articulating the right to transnational practices. Article 36 (1) states, "Indigenous peoples, in particular those divided by interna-tional borders, have the right to maintain and develop contacts, relations and cooperation, including activities for spiritual, cultural, political, eco-nomic and social purposes, with their own members as well as peoples across borders" (UN General Assembly 2007).

Clearly, transnational organising, networking, lobbying, and advocacy are essential practices for social, economic, and political transformation. While the human rights agenda can be used to contest and appeal current life cir-cumstances and create avenues to challenge the constitutionality of structural discrepancies and inequities and make demands for redress and compensation, the individualistic focus has been critiqued from an Aboriginal perspective that generally supports a more collectivist, interdependent ontology. A difficulty with international treaties is the inability to hold nations accountable, even when they are signatories. As Clayton Thomas Muller of the Mathais Colomb Cree Nation, Tar Sands Campaign organiser for the Indigenous Environmen-tal Network, recently claimed, "Canada is the only country still opposing the UN Declaration on the Rights of Indigenous Peoples. Canada continues to criminalize Indigenous activists who stand up for Aboriginal Treaty rights, even though these rights have been affirmed by the Canadian constitution and the UN Declaration on the Rights of Indigenous Peoples" (Thomas Muller 2010). This state opposition was finally overturned in November 2010 with Canada's endorsement of the UN Declaration. In the case of state opposition, or lack of implementation through a system of protections and sanctions, recourse leads to appeals through international coalitions, and the activation of pressures applied both on the global stage and domestically.

Indigenous peoples have also organised effectively to tackle transna-tional environmental concerns. The land and, more specifically, a commu-nity's sacred relationship with the land (Little Bear 1998; Wilson 2008) have always been a source of cultural identity for Indigenous peoples. Envi-ronmental degradation, including air and water pollution, land contamina-tion, soil erosion, desertification, natural resource depletion, and global warming, as well as the appropriation and marketisation of Indigenous knowledge and medicinal plants, have become the new form of 'ecological imperialism.' In the time of imperial and colonial expansion, western Euro-peans brought what Crosby (1986) termed a "portmanteau biota" com-plete with plants, animals, and pathogens that made possible European numerical supremacy in the "land of the demographic takeover." Now it is industrialised nations and their degrading land-use practices, polluting industrial and technological processes, that constitute present-day ecological imperialism in the manner of transboundary air pollution, diminished ability to engage in traditional land-use practices, environmental refugees, and so on. Just as the social, cultural, historical, and economic boundaries of nation-states are fluid, so too are environmental boundaries, often with the worst offenses by industrial nations accruing to those communities not participating in their production or enjoying their benefits.

A clear statement of the profound connection Indigenous peoples have with their land base is expressed in a letter to U.S. Senator John Kerry composed by youth representing Athabasca Chipewyan First Nation, Beaver Lake Cree First Nation, and Lubicon Cree First Nation regarding the devastation caused by the Alberta oil sands. Fearing that Canadian Environment Minister Jim Prentice would downplay the significant human rights and environmental iniquities of the oil sands when meeting with U.S. Congressional leaders, the youth wrote: "Animals are dying, disappearing, and being mutated by the poisons dumped into our river systems. . . . Once we have destroyed these fragile eco-systems we will have also destroyed our peoples and trampled our treaty rights" (Indigenous Environmental Network (IEN) 2009).

In response to the disproportionate environmental risks Indigenous peoples face nationally and globally, Indigenous environmental activists have formed transnational coalitions, networks, and organisations, sometimes working in concert with non-Indigenous nongovernmental organisations to combat environmental racism, terminate environmental wrongs, and seek remediation. One need only reflect on the dire environmental conditions experienced in Aamjiwnaang First Nation in southern Ontario or the Cree and Chipewyan First Nations in Alberta to comprehend the extent of environmental injustices within Canadian borders (Nikiforuk 2008).[5] Internationally, the differential exposure to environmental carcinogens and neurotoxins experienced by Indigenous peoples is meticulously documented by Westra (2007). The Indigenous Environmental Network, which has a twenty-year history, for example, has been working to promote environmental justice and sustainable livelihoods in First Nations communities, addressing issues such as climate change, environmental toxins, biodiversity, sacred places, water concerns, and globalisation.

The Inuit Circumpolar Council (ICC), another Indigenous transnational coalition, comprises Inuit from Canada, Russia, Alaska, and Greenland, and serves to protect Inuit human, cultural, and language rights, as well as safeguard the Arctic environment for present and future generations. The ICC played a substantial role in the international negotiations that led to ratifying the Stockholm Convention on the Elimination of Persistent Organic Pollutants, a convention that came into force in 2003. These are but a few examples, among many, of Indigenous peoples employing transnational processes and avenues to make significant assertions regarding environmental, human, and social justice rights.

NORTHERN RESOURCE DEVELOPMENT—
FIRST NATIONS AND CANADA

Much of the transnational literature has examined the practices, dynamics, and social and societal impacts of persons moving from poorer to wealthier nations, the flow of transnational labour created by migrants who seek economic opportunities that will permit greater material provisions, through remittances sent from the host country to family members back home (Crawford 2003; Parreñas 2005; Beck-Gernsheim 2007; Cornelius et al. 2009). Immigrants, refugees, and asylum seekers have been considered in diasporic, transnational analyses, but not Aboriginal peoples and their movements within Canadian borders, despite the fact that Aboriginal peoples define their communities as separate nations contained within the historical imposed boundaries delineating the geographic and political purview of Canada. Movements outside of First Nations borders represent a form of transnationalism, and this section will demonstrate how these flows, when stemming from economic incentives, show many of the hallmarks of transnational practices globally.

Transmigrants often experience a considerable economic difference between their home and prospective host countries, which acts as an inducement for transnational strivings (Beck-Gernsheim 2007). It is precisely these kinds of flows in human labour that are investigated in transnational scholarship, in situations where the divide between rich and poor is so severe that families will tolerate lengthy geographic separations for the sake of alleviating this economic gap. Just over a decade ago, Aboriginal peoples were described as enduring some of the most deplorable living conditions within Canadian borders: ill health, poverty, contaminated water, dilapidated and overcrowded housing, and family breakdown (Indian and Northern Affairs Canada 2000). This report likened the experiences of Aboriginal peoples to those of people living in 'Third World' countries. The analogy, based on the statistical evidence, is apt and invokes Manuel's (1974) use of the designation 'Fourth World' to signal the economic, political, and social disparities separating the so-called First World from Indigenous peoples' Fourth World conditions. More recent statistics indicate Aboriginal peoples in Canada fared poorer than the general population on a variety of health indices, including diabetes, heart disease, and addiction (Health Canada 2009), showing significantly higher rates of suicide (Government of Canada 2006). And, irrespective of subtle improvements in Aboriginal employment rates from 2001 to 2006, these rates remain considerably below those of the average figures for the general Canadian population, with on-reserve Aboriginal groups having even higher unemployment rates than their counterparts who live off reserve (Statistics Canada 2009).

Given these statistics, it is not surprising that the Aboriginal practice of rural- or reserve-urban migration, in which individuals leave their First Nation to enter large urban centres, is often motivated by ambitions not dissimilar to those of non-Aboriginal transmigrants. While some Aboriginal persons endeavour primarily to escape the poverty or terrible circumstances of their home community, what some have termed 'rural ghettoes' (Dei, Hall, and Rosenberg 2000: 9), others leave their home community, their First Nation, and venture into the larger social and political topography of the Canadian nation-state to achieve improved material standards, present and future, for themselves and their extended families (Mt. Pleasant, personal communication, 21 July 2010). This form of transnational movement shares many parallels with transnational practices in the larger global context, replete with remittances to family members at home, use of information and communication technologies to sustain long-distance ties, dual consciousness and the bifocality of being here and there, lesser economic and social status in the host country, and, sometimes, family breakdown.

The shift in the past quarter century from a world economy having international practices to a global market characterised by transnational forces and increasing fluidity of nation-state borders engendering altered and accelerated patterns of human, information, capital, and corporate flows is impacting Indigenous peoples in multiple, and sometimes unambiguously negative ways (Hall and Fenelon 2009). This is especially true when considering top-down transnational manoeuvrings of the growing corporate-state, the very practices that the transnationalism 'from below,' both as ambition for increased prosperity and radical equity praxis, seeks to mitigate (Morawska 2003). Globalisation processes in the Canadian context must be explored for their unique effects on Aboriginal peoples and their communities. In this time of neoliberal market developments the Canadian government is more strongly supporting Aboriginal self-governance, which should not be hastily interpreted as progress, for this change in political tone cannot be read separate from growing industry interests in Aboriginal territories now known to be resource-rich (Slowey 2001). In the past, Canadian developments on Crown lands [6] bypassed consultations with Aboriginal peoples, but in recent decades the negotiated agreement, signalling an evolution in First Nations-corporate relations, is central to resource development in First Nations Treaty areas. This change has been achieved largely through Aboriginal resistance and political activism and the consequent changes in legislation and the *Constitution Act*. The relatively recent discovery of mineral-rich areas in the boreal region of Canada, most of them on Aboriginal Treaty lands, has led to a growing number of negotiated agreements between First Nations and corporations throughout subarctic Canada.

The unsettling unemployment rates and health statistics already discussed coupled with the significant labour market barriers Aboriginal peoples face because of discrimination, lower education levels, and limited job opportunities near their home communities (Luffman and Sussman 2007) make these negotiated agreements, essentially a First Nation-corporate agreement, appealing. Unfortunately these new economic developments, while potentially a boon to the local First Nations economies, are not entirely without unpromising social consequences. While the incomes of those working at the mines are generally high and each First Nation usually negotiates the right of its members to have first opportunity for jobs, the actual work schedule is often gruelling, typically involving two-week rotations where employees fly into the remote region where the mine is situated, are away from their families half the month, which cumulatively amounts to half the year (Dylan, Smallboy, and Lightman, in progress). In the transnational space, or "diaspora space" (Brah 1996), of the mine site tenuously 'inhabited' by Aboriginal peoples from various First Nations as well as non-Aboriginal persons, in the association of multiple cultural identities, lies the potentiality for new transnational subjectivities. Family breakdown sometimes occurs as absence strains fidelity. Sometimes couples decide to move out of their First Nation and into the closest town, even while one partner continues to fly back and forth to the mine, because they wish to avail themselves of educational opportunities and the more affordable material goods in these non-Aboriginal centres (Dylan et al., in progress). Although this form of Aboriginal transnationalism has not been sufficiently studied, the risks to the social fabric, cultural values, and traditional lifeways (stemming in part from the environmental damage caused by mining practices) are considerable, yet so is the persistent cost of poverty, as so many statistics for Aboriginal peoples in Canada demonstrate.

Some of these issues could be addressed through creating meaningful participation opportunities for all parties in the negotiation process (Stewart and Sinclair 2007), seeking and suitably considering traditional ecological knowledge to help sustain traditional lands (Whitelaw, McCarthy, and Tsuji 2009; Mulvihill and Baker 2001; Armitage 2005), and militating against the cultural and power disparities of proponents and stakeholders by insisting on just negotiations as a starting point (Banerjee 2000; Chataway 2002). These issues ought to be considered in a transnational context, in the nation-to-nation and transnational framework of global and local concerns, if they are to be properly and equitably addressed.

## CONCLUDING COMMENTS

We started from the absence of Aboriginal realities in discussions of transnationalism. We examined some of the reasons and circumstances for this absence and presented three cases of transnational relations in which Aboriginal peoples were central, which can extend the parameters of what transnational relations encompass. We hope to have shown some of the specificities, as well as some commonalities of Indigenous transnational experiences with current understandings of transnational relations: first, cultural influences and shifting patterns during pre-Confederation situations of transnational relations that were motivated by economic gains for the settler powers, which have been devalued and are more difficult to document; second, recent networking of Indigenous peoples across national borders for purposes of activism in the making of joint claims addressed to nation-states and the forces of the neoliberal market through international organisations; and third, within the borders of a nation-state (a case that is typically left out of transnational considerations), a transnational type of relations between and across Indigenous communities and mainstream society as found in a local economic venture. Economics, cultures, and relations of power are at stake, and are negotiated through daily personal contacts.

Each of these discussions has brought out a different facet of the kind of social support that is at stake in varied circumstances. The early historical case, which suggested a form of co-existence on a daily basis that led to forms of exchange, support, and hybridisation across peoples, was subsumed under other power relations, making the traces of inter-group support very tenuous. To lift those early realities into our awareness would require a particular type of scholarship focusing on the unheard voices of secondary (perhaps mediating) social actors. The second configuration of the global alliances illustrates the formidable development of formal mechanisms of mutual support and empowerment developed conjointly by Aboriginal nations in their dealings with non-Aboriginal nations. The third type of circumstance strongly suggests the need for the participatory involvement of Aboriginal people in the type of economic decision-making that affects communities, beyond the interests of the market and the short-term assistance to specific individuals. These strategies are not exhaustive.

The objective in this chapter was to engage with the broader question of the absence of Aboriginal realities in debates on transnationalism, and the cases discussed are illustrations that cover a particular spectrum of processes. Other sets of questions, situations, or circumstances could be examined beyond these specific instances. In preparing this chapter, other paths of inquiry came to mind, which we offer as a sample among possible others.

Instances of transnationalism among Indigenous peoples abound. Historically, in the case of the American continent, Indigenous people have felt connected across the borders of the nation-states that are now Canada, the U.S., and the formerly French, Spanish, and English colonies. People travelled back and forth along the north-south lines, and maintained concrete, personal, family, and community ties. The notion of time being more elastic and stretching over much longer periods for Aboriginal peoples also means that such communities' ties can be relationally and symbolically maintained for extensive periods of time. In fact, border crossing is an imposition from the nation-states, which is thought of instead as land continuity that goes back to pre-colonial times. The state partitions are relatively recent and do not coincide with people's practices even today. This line of investigation would encompass the actual practices of settlement, various forms of mobility, visitation, celebrations, and exchanges between individuals, families, and members of community across the nation-state borders.

A related but different question which links to this point, and also to the second case we discussed in terms of alliances, is that Indigenous peoples across North, Central, and South America have maintained an interest in the well-being of Indigenous peoples 'on the other side' of that border. The realities of their comparable fates within settler states resulting from colonialism has naturally generated a sense of common interests and common concern for the welfare and conversely the dislocation of Indigenous communities across the continent, and the value placed on Indigenous values and knowledge. Such a line of inquiry would pursue the symbolic affiliations across Indigenous communities that have been developed for cultural, social, and political ends.

Some of the Indigenous-settler state relations have been marked by a long history of legal disputations. Numerous examples abound, as mentioned early on in our chapter. The terms of these legal arrangements and their implementation would lend themselves to close examination. This is a type of scholarship that is currently removed from discussions of transnationalism, although this concern implicates the rewriting of a public history (Johnson 2008). A case in point is the Jay Treaty of 1794 signed between the two colonial powers of the time, the British Crown and the U.S., without Aboriginal peoples being signatories to it. The treaty recognises the Aboriginal right of mobility of people and commodities across the newly constituted borders without interference, e.g., without taxation, penalty, or hindrance. It provides the right for status-Aboriginal peoples (defined by evidence of Aboriginal blood quantum greater than 50 percent) to enter the U.S. without a passport; the right to be employed in the U.S. without requiring a special work permit (such as the green card). This treaty is still in force, yet it is known to some Aboriginal peoples and is invisible to most people. The extent of its applicability today would be a significant path of inquiry. The meaning of its existence, which once affirmed the primacy of Aboriginal peoples' rights to the land and resources, has most likely been eroded.

The many cultural and symbolic connections across Indigenous peoples lend themselves to a wide range of investigations in the arenas of culture, communication, and the arts. Different generations of Indigenous peoples have maintained and produced cultural and spiritual works, which in turn have had different kinds of imprints and influences among different audiences. Inquiries need to be made into the institutional arrangements that have sustained such creations, and into the obstacles to their maintenance and expansion, the extent and density of the networks and media affiliations. Examining current productions would constitute another stimulating avenue of study; for example, in what ways do urban Aboriginal theatre productions transmit, negotiate, and work with transnational realities among Indigenous groups and in relation to mainstream or minority productions?

Many questions of concern to Aboriginal peoples can be thought of in transnational terms. We feel strongly about the importance of including Aboriginal realities in the agenda of transnationalism. We hope to have shown, at least in a preliminary manner, particular instances of such processes, and how their specificities can extend our understandings of transnational realities.

## NOTES

1. The *Calder v. British Columbia (Attorney General)* decision represented the first acknowledgement in Canadian law that Aboriginal title, and rights to land, existed before and persist following colonisation. This decision initiated the readiness of the federal government to negotiate First Nations land claims.
2. In the Supreme Court of Canada ruling on *Delgamuukw v. British Columbia* the parameters of Aboriginal title, its content and extent, were further defined. This ruling acknowledges rights to specified lands belonging to Aboriginal peoples, provided that exclusive use and occupation can be demonstrated continuing since the British Crown declared dominion over the territory. This case also led to the ruling that Aboriginal peoples' oral histories were to be recognised as evidence when establishing historic occupation or use.
3. This term refers to lands thought to belong to Aboriginal peoples based on rights deriving from formal agreements established in treaties between sovereign nations: Aboriginal nations and the Crown.
4. The Indian Act is the primary federal statute regarding Aboriginal (Indian) status, governance, and management of lands. It has been rightly decried by Aboriginal peoples as paternalistic, colonial, and detrimental to self-government.
5. Both the Aamjiwnaang First Nation and the Cree and Chipewyan First Nations are suffering health problems caused by environmental contaminants. For Aamjiwnaang residents the source is more than sixty industrial facilities, by which the nation is surrounded, releasing staggering levels of toxic industrial byproducts into the environment; for Cree and Chipewyan First Nations in Alberta, it is environmental toxins produced by the oil sands.
6. The term Crown lands refers to those lands owned by the provincial or federal governments. Based on relevant Supreme Court rulings regarding Aboriginal title, if the government desires to pursue any activity on Crown land, a reasonable attempt must be made to determine whether Aboriginal rights exist, and if they do, the Aboriginal nations holding these rights must be consulted.

## BIBLIOGRAPHY

Alia, V. (2010) *The New Media Nation: Indigenous Peoples and Global Communication*. New York: Berghahn Books.

Armitage, D. (2005) 'Collaborative Environmental Assessment in the Northwest Territories, Canada.' *Environmental Impact Assessment Review*, 25(3): 239–58.

Banerjee, S. B. (2000) 'Whose Land Is It Anyway? National Interest, Indigenous Stakeholders, and Colonial Discourses.' *Organization & Environment*, 13(1): 3–39.

Beck-Gernsheim, E. (2007) 'Transnational Lives, Transnational Marriages: A Review of the Evidence from Migrant Communities in Europe.' *Global Networks*, 7(3): 271–88.

Becker, A. E., R. A. Burwell, and S. E. Gilman (2002) 'Eating Behaviours and Attitudes following Prolonged Exposure to Television among Ethnic Fijian Adolescent Girls.' *The British Journal of Psychiatry*, 180: 509–14.

Biggar, H. P. (1922–36) *The Works of Samuel de Champlain*. 6 vols. Toronto: The Champlain Society.

Brah, A. (1996) *Cartographies of Diaspora: Contesting Identities*. London and New York: Routledge.

Cardinal, H. (1999) *The Unjust Society: The Tragedy of Canada's Indians*. Reprint. Toronto: Douglas & McIntyre Publishers, Inc.

Chataway, C. (2002) 'Successful Development in Aboriginal Communities: Does It Depend upon a Particular Process?' *The Journal of Aboriginal Economic Development*, 3(1): 76–88.

Christie, G. (2005) 'A Colonial Reading of Recent Jurisprudence: Sparrow, Delgamuukw and Haifa Nation.' *Windsor Yearbook of Access to Justice*, 23: 17–53. http://papers.ssrn.com/sol13/papers.cfm?abstrct_id=1636029. Retrieved 17 September 2010.

Coates, K. (2004) *A Global History of Indigenous Peoples: Struggle and Survival*. New York: Palgrave Macmillan.

Cornelius, W. A., D. Fitzgerald, J. Hernandez-Diaz, and S. Borger, eds. (2009) *Migration from the Mexican Mixteca: A Transnational Community in Oaxaca and California*. San Diego: University of California, Center for Comparative Immigration Studies.

Crawford, C. (2003) 'Sending Love in a Barrel: The Making of Transnational Caribbean Families in Canada.' *Canadian Women Studies*, 22(3/4): 104–9.

Crosby, A. (1986) *Ecological Imperialism: The Biological Expansion of Europe, 900–1900*. New York: Cambridge University Press.

de Costa, R. (2006) *A Higher Authority: Indigenous Transnationalism and Australia*. Sydney: University of New South Wales.

Dei, G. J. S., B. L. Hall, and D. G. Rosenberg (2000) 'Introduction.' In *Indigenous Knowledges in Global Contexts: Multiple Readings of Our World*, edited by G. J. S. Dei, B. L. Hall, and D. G. Rosenberg, 3–17. Toronto: University of Toronto Press.

Dickason, O. P. (1993) 'Jus Gentium Takes on New Meanings.' In *The Law of Nations and the New World*, edited by L. C. Green and O. P. Dickason, 227–240. Edmonton, AB: University of Alberta Press.

Dickason, O. P. (2002) *Canada's First Nations: A History of Founding Peoples from the Earliest Times*. 3rd ed. Don Mills, ON: Oxford University Press.

Dylan, A., B. Smallboy, and E. Lightman (in progress) '"Saying No to Resource Development Is Not an Option": Economic Development in Moose Cree First Nation.'

Faulstich Orellana, M., B. Thorne, A. Chee, and W. S. E. Lam (2001) 'Transnational Childhoods: The Participation of Children in Processes of Family Migration.' *Social Problems*, 48(4): 572–91.

Government of Canada (2006) 'The Mental Health and Well-Being of Aboriginal Peoples in Canada.' In *The Human Face of Mental Health and Mental Illness in Canada*, 159–80. Ottawa: Minister of Public Works and Government Services Canada.

Hall, T. D., and J. B. Fenelon (2009) *Indigenous Peoples and Globalization: Resistance and Revitalization*. Boulder: Paradigm Publishers.

Health Canada (2009) *A Statistical Profile on the Health of First Nations in Canada: Determinants of Health 1999 to 2003*. Ottawa: Health Canada.

Henderson Youngblood, J. (Sákéj) (2000) '*Ayukpachi*: Empowering Aboriginal Thought.' In *Reclaiming Indigenous Voice and Vision*, edited by M. Battiste, 248–278. Vancouver and Toronto: UBC Press.

Hobsbawm, E. J. (1990) *Nations and Nationalism since 1780: Programme, Myth, Reality*. 2nd ed. Cambridge: Cambridge University Press.

Hondagneu-Sotelo, P., and E. Avila (1997) '"I'm Here, but I'm There": The Meanings of Latina Transnational Motherhood.' *Gender and Society*, 11(5): 548–71.

Indian and Northern Affairs Canada [INAC] (2000) *Gathering Strength: Canada's Aboriginal Action Plan, A Progress Report.* Ottawa: Department of Indian Affairs and Northern Development.

Indigenous Environmental Network (2009) 'Canadian Environment Minister Preempted by First Nation Youth.' http://www.ienearth.org/tarsands.html. Retrieved 6 June 2010.

Johnson, M. (2008) 'Making History Public: Indigenous Claims to Settler States.' *Public Culture*, 20(1): 97–117.

Landolt, P. (2001) 'Salvadoran Economic Transnationalism: Embedded Strategies for Household Maintenance, Immigrant Incorporation, and Entrepreneurial Expansion.' *Global Networks*, 1(3): 217–41.

Le Clercq, C. (1691) *Premier Etablissement de la Foy dans la Nouvelle-France.* 2 vols. Paris: A. Auroy.

Levitt, P., and N. Glick Schiller (2004) 'Conceptualizing Simultaneity: A Transnational Social Field Perspective on Society.' *International Migration Review*, 38(3): 1002–39.

Little Bear, L. (1998) 'Aboriginal Relationships to the Land and Resources.' In *Sacred Lands: Aboriginal World Views, Claims and Conflicts*, edited by J. Oakes, R. Riewe, K. Kinew, and E. Maloney, 15–20. Edmonton: Canadian Circumpolar Institute and Department of Native Studies.

Lorde, A. (1984) *Sister Outsider: Essays and Speeches by Audre Lorde.* Berkeley: Crossing Press.

Luffman, J., and D. Sussman (2007) 'The Aboriginal Labour Force in Western Canada.' *Perspectives on Labour and Income*, 19(1): 30–44.

Mander, J. (1991) *In the Absence of the Sacred: The Failure of Technology and the Survival of the Indian Nations.* San Francisco: Sierra Club Books.

Manuel, G. (1974) *The Fourth World: An Indian Reality.* Don Mills, ON: Collier-Macmillan.

Miller, J. R. (2000) *Skyscrapers Hide the Heavens: A History of Indian-White Relations in Canada.* 3rd ed. Toronto: University of Toronto Press.

Morawska, E. (2003) 'Disciplinary Agendas and Analytic Strategies of Research on Immigrant Transnationalism: Challenges of Interdisciplinary Knowledge.' *International Migration Review*, 37(3): 611–40.

Mulvihill, P. R., and D. C. Baker (2001) 'Ambitious and Restrictive Scoping: Case Studies from Northern Canada.' *Environmental Impact Assessment Review*, 21: 363–84.

Nikiforuk, A. (2008) *Tar Sands: Dirty Oil and the Future of a Continent.* Vancouver: Greystone Books.

Paehlke, R. C. (2004) *Democracy's Dilemma: Environment, Social Equity, and the Global Economy.* Cambridge, MA: The MIT Press.

Parrenas, R. S. (2005) *Children of Global Migration: Transnational Families and Gendered Woes.* Palo Alto: Stanford University Press.

Persky, S. (1998) *Delgamuukw: The Supreme Court of Canada Decision on Aboriginal Title.* Vancouver: Greystone Books.

Royal Commission on Aboriginal Peoples [RCAP] (1996) *People to People, Nation to Nation: Highlights from the Report of the Royal Commission on Aboriginal Peoples.* Ottawa: Minister of Supply and Services Canada.

Sagard, G. (1866) *Histoire du Canada et voyages que les frères mineurs récollects y ont faicts pour la conversion des infidèles depuis l'an 1615.* 4 vols. Paris: Edwin Tross.

Said, E. (1994) *Culture and Imperialism.* New York: Vintage Books.

Sayre, R. (2008) *La Modernité et Son Autre. Récits de la Rencontre avec l'Indien en Amérique du Nord au XVIIIe siècle.* Bécherel: Les Perséides.
Slowey, G. (2001) 'Globalization and Self-Government: Impacts and Implications for First Nations in Canada.' *American Review of Canadian Studies*, 31(1/2): 265–81.
Spivak, G. C. (1990) *The Post-Colonial Critic: Interviews, Strategies, Dialogues.* New York: Routledge.
Statistics Canada (2007) *Canada Year Book, 2007: Aboriginal Peoples.* Ottawa: Statistics Canada. http://www.41.statcan.ca/2007/10000/ceb10000_0_e.htm. Retrieved 6 June 2010.
Statistics Canada (2009) *Labour Force Historical Review, 2008.* Ottawa: Statistics Canada. http://www4.hrsdc.gc.ca/.3ndic.1t.4r@-eng.jsp?iid=16. Retrieved 4 June 2010.
Stewart, J., and J. Sinclair (2007) 'Meaningful Public Participation in Environmental Assessment: Perspectives from Canadian Participants, Proponents, and Government.' *Journal of Environmental Assessment Policy and Management*, 9(2): 161–83.
Thomas Muller, C. (2010) 'Canada Can't Hide Genocide.' Talk given at the 'Shout Out' (G8/G20) Day of Action, Toronto, 24 June 2010.
Thwaites, R. G., ed. (1896–1901) *The Jesuit Relations and Allied Documents.* 73 vols. Cleveland: Burrows Brothers.
Tinsman, H., and S. Shukla (2007) 'Introduction: Across the Americas.' In *Imagining Our Americas: Toward a Transnational Frame*, edited by H. Tinsman and S. Shukla, 1–25. Durham and London: Duke University Press.
Trigger, B. (1987) *The Children of Aataentsic: A History of the Huron People to 1660.* Kingston and Montreal: McGill-Queen's University Press.
Trigger, B. (1994) *Natives and Newcomers: Canada's "Heroic Age" Reconsidered.* Montreal: McGill-Queen's University Press.
UN General Assembly (2007) Resolution 61/295, 'United Nations Declaration on the Rights of Indigenous Peoples.' 13 September 2007. Audiovisual Library of International Law, http://untreaty.un.org/cod/avl/ha/ga_61–295.html. Retrieved 17 September 2010.
Vertovec, S. (1999) 'Conceiving and Researching Transnationalism.' *Ethnic and Racial Studies*, 22: 447–62.
Vertovec, S. (2004) 'Migrant Transnationalism and Modes of Transformation.' *International Migration Review*, 38(3): 970–1001.
Westra, L. (2007) *Environmental Justice and the Rights of Indigenous Peoples: International and Domestic Legal Perspectives.* London: Earthscan.
Whitelaw, G. S., D. D. McCarthy, and L. J. S. Tsuji (2009) 'The Victor Diamond Mine Environmental Assessment Process: A Critical First Nation Perspective.' *Impact Assessment and Project Appraisal*, 27(3): 205–15.
Wilson, S. (2008) *Research Is Ceremony: Indigenous Research Methods.* Black Point, NS: Fernwood Publishing.
Wimmer, A., and N. Glick Schiller (2003) 'Transnational Migration: International Perspectives.' *International Migration Review*, 37(3): 576–610.
Wolf, E. [1982] (1997) *Europe and the People without History.* 2nd printing. Berkeley: University of California Press.
Wrong, G. M. (1939) *The Long Journey to the Country of the Hurons.* Toronto: The Champlain Society.

# 11 Paradoxes of Transnational Knowledge Production in Social Work

*Stefan Köngeter*

## INTRODUCTION

Transnational studies pose a challenge to social work that is reflected on at least two distinct levels. First, there is growing evidence that social relations and practices cannot be analysed only within the confines of the nation-state anymore, as numerous transnational processes can be observed that transcend those confines at the level of individuals, communities, or organisations. Second, the debate about the transnationalisation of the social world (Pries 2008) shows that the neglect of these transnational processes is a symptom of an inherent weakness in social science methodology and theory building. The social sciences have overlooked the importance and the changing meaning of the nation, the nation-state, and its institutions, e.g., territory, law, or authority (Sassen 2008). This blind spot, referred to as methodological nationalism (Wimmer and Glick Schiller 2002), has hindered the exploration of transnational processes already underway for some time.

This chapter is based on the assumption that social work is also affected by methodological nationalism (section 2). My argument does not, however, take up the proposal to develop a transnational methodology, as for example in the work of Khagram and Levitt (2008). Instead, a sociology of scientific knowledge informed by post-colonialism and feminism is taken as a basis for the argument that knowledge production itself should be examined and deconstructed, which, in turn, would enable us to find vital clues about the development of methodological nationalism (section 3). After an overview of previous research into the transnational production of knowledge in social work (section 4), the case study of the settlement movement is introduced (section 5). Alix Westerkamp's "Letters from American Settlements" (1917–19) represents an early example of transnational knowledge production (section 6) which is not only historically significant for social work because of the settlement movement, but draws attention to paradoxical phenomena within a transnational production of knowledge (section 7).

## THE METHODOLOGICAL NATIONALISM
## OF THE SOCIAL SCIENCES

As a result of growing concern with the phenomena of globalisation (Beck 2000), the transnationalisation of the social world (Glick Schiller, Basch, and Blanc-Szanton 1992), and the global diffusion of western culture (Meyer 2009), social science theory and methodology are faced with the central challenge of determining what significance the nation-state and its institutions still have. Theories of transnationality, cosmopolitanism, or globalisation criticise an unreflective and inadequate approach to the nation and the nation-state. Both classical and current sociological theories are accused of fostering *methodological nationalism*, which is described as an anachronistic, and largely implicit, assumption about social reality: "Methodological nationalism considers nation states as the basic unit of all politics. It assumes that humankind is naturally distributed among a limited number of nations, which organise themselves internally as nation states and delimit themselves externally from other nation states" (Zürn 2003: 358).[1]

The most comprehensive and detailed criticism of methodological nationalism was developed by Wimmer and Glick Schiller (2002), who identified a problematic isomorphism of national-state institutions and schemes of analysis in the field of social sciences. Wimmer and Glick Schiller distinguish three forms of methodological nationalism. Especially in what they call sociological "grand theories," i.e., the grand theories of the sociological classics such as Max Weber and Talcott Parsons, the importance of the nation-state as one of the key principles of modernity is largely *ignored*. This underestimation of the importance and persistence of the nation-state prevents a deeper analysis of the transformations of nationalism, the nation-state, and its institutions. A second variant consists of the *naturalisation* or *reification* of a nation-state perspective. In political science, economics, anthropology, etc., nation-state–oriented categories were used as the unquestioned framework for analysis; social processes within the nation-state are, as a matter of course, distinguished from processes outside, without realising that and how they relate to each other. Finally, a third form of methodological nationalism, i.e., the hypostasis of territorial border creation, has been met with criticism. The social sciences are accused of painting a picture of the nation-state and society as a container, in which a clearly defined territory confines culture, politics, economy, and community.

According to their argumentation, these three different variants of methodological nationalism mutually reinforce each other and are represented to different degrees in the respective sub-disciplines of the social sciences: while the so-called grand theories largely ignore nationalism and the nation-state, they are reified or naturalised in the empirically oriented social sciences and are territorialised in historical studies.[2]

It is not the aim of this chapter to show whether social work also follows narrow conceptions of the nation-state and the welfare state. An analysis of the methodological nationalism of social work in Germany has already been undertaken elsewhere (Köngeter 2009). This analysis shows that theories in social work often use a concept of society without adequately stressing the relationship between the term 'society' and the persisting importance of the nation-state. As it is not made explicit to what extent this nation-state and its welfare institutions continue to shape social reality, the nation-state remains a commonsensical, quasi-natural, and pragmatic angle in social work. The implicit nature of the nation-state is strengthened by the fact that research, as well as its funding institutions, also refer as a matter of course to fields of activity whose boundaries are determined by welfare-state institutions. The productions of welfare and of scholarship are in large part shaped by the nation-state and, therefore, reinforce the national framework of each other.

It would be inadequate, however, merely to argue for a transnational production of knowledge and methodology (Khagram and Levitt 2008). This approach would mean, first of all, missing the opportunity to discover those attempts at transnational knowledge production and methodology which already exist. Furthermore, it would mean taking up an epistemologically problematic position: criticising the social sciences and their methodology from an external standpoint, as it were, without reflecting on the fact that the critique itself is also a part of this discursive context.

## DECONSTRUCTING METHODOLOGICAL NATIONALISM

A perspective informed by feminism, post-colonialism, and the sociology of scientific knowledge takes a fundamentally different position. Within this theoretical context, knowledge in academia is principally seen as "situated knowledge" (Clifford 1989; Haraway 1991). The social sciences and their theories cannot claim to describe social reality from the outside, but rather, each description as part of social reality is anchored *in* a social reality. With Pierre Bourdieu one can demand that, because of "the inextricable relationship of scientific—and hence also sociological—practice with overall societal competition and struggle for power, sociology has to turn these facts into an object of its own research, i.e., the tools of science have to be applied to science itself" (Eickelpasch 2002: 57).

From such a reflexive perspective, one's own framework of academic production has to be addressed critically. Such a perspective from the sociology of knowledge is therefore not content with diagnosing that there is (at least the tendency of) a largely hidden nation-state bias in the production of knowledge and theory in social work, but it would inquire into the factors and conditions of its emergence. This approach not only gives rise to a methodological discussion in transnational studies, but also opens up a new field of research with numerous questions which have rarely been taken into consideration to date, and which have not been adequately investigated either for the social sciences or for social work.

This chapter assumes a primarily historical perspective on the research field of (trans)national knowledge production. The questions arising from this point of view include: how has the development of social work been influenced by knowledge from other national contexts? Along what routes has knowledge in social work spread transnationally? What contextualisations and transformations have been accomplished? To what extent have such processes in social work increased awareness of transnational phenomena, possible solutions, and theoretical reflections? When and how did a narrow methodological nationalism come to prevail?

When it comes to reconstructing these questions, there are certain important starting points, in addition to the fundamental considerations of Bourdieu outlined earlier. A striking example of this is Said's study (1983), in which he traces the transformation undergone by Lukács's theory of reification. Said analyses how this theory was adopted by Lukács's student Goldmann (1973) and later by the Welsh literary scholar Williams (1973), who ultimately utilised this Goldmann-Lukács theory for his literary studies. Said (1983: 238) offers a critical summary:

> Without wishing in any way to belittle the importance of what Lukacs' ideas (via Goldmann) did for the moribund state of English studies in late twentieth-century Cambridge, I think it needs to be said that those ideas were originally formulated in order to do more than shake up a few professors of literature. This is an obvious, not to say easy, point. What is more interesting, however, is that because Cambridge is not revolutionary Budapest, because Williams is not the militant Lukacs, because Williams is a reflective critic—this is crucial—rather than a committed revolutionary, he can see the limits of a theory that begins as a liberating idea but can become a trap of its own.

This example points to the general conditions for a 'travelling theory.' Said works on the assumption of a multi-stage model, according to which a theory first arises from a particular set of conditions, then it travels a certain distance in space and time, where it is confronted with new conditions and is therefore adapted and transformed (Said 1983: 227). Clifford (1989) takes up this idea and radicalises it. He argues that Said's concept of the ways theories are transformed is too simple. Instead he returns to the Greek roots of the word and paraphrases theories as "a practice of travel and observation, a man sent by the polis to another city to witness a religious ceremony" (Clifford 1989: para. 1). He concludes from this that theory is an act of displacement, distancing, and comparison. Theorising thus means leaving one's native country, going abroad, but also returning home with new knowledge. Yet at the same time he objects that such a concept of home no longer exists in the post-colonial age:

> Theory is no longer naturally 'at home' in the West—a powerful place of Knowledge, History, or Science, a place to collect, sift, translate, and

generalise. Or, more cautiously, this privileged place is now increasingly contested, cut across, by other locations, claims, trajectories of knowledge articulating racial, gender, and cultural differences. But how is theory appropriated and resisted, located and displaced? How do theories travel among the unequal spaces of postcolonial confusion and contestation? What are their predicaments? How does theory travel and how do theorists travel? Complex, unresolved questions. (Clifford 1989: para. 8)

The diffusion and circulation of knowledge and ideas have attracted greater attention in the context of the increasing preoccupation, in the social sciences, with phenomena of globalisation and transnationalisation. Surprisingly, transnational studies play only a small role in this context. Instead, neo-institutional studies[3] (Hasse and Krücken 2005) are partly responsible for drawing attention to these boundary-crossing forms of knowledge production (Meyer 2009). The early neo-institutional investigations, however, do not clarify which practices make the diffusion of this knowledge possible or how the knowledge is transformed (Sahlin and Wedlin 2008). Another important approach for studying the circulation of ideas is that of the laboratory studies of Latour, Callon, and others (Latour and Woolgar 1979; Callon 1980), which, with the aid of the concept of *translation*, open up a microanalytical perspective. This makes it possible to show that, despite transnational and global tendencies to homogenisation, the transfer of knowledge from one social world to another (Star and Griesemer 1989; Strauss 1993) is always associated with a transformation, which is fundamentally undefined and open (Callon 1980).

## TRAVELLING THEORY IN SOCIAL WORK

Let us now turn to the question of how, in the history of social work,[4] knowledge, ideas and theories have circulated, left their own nation-state contexts, and been received in others. Little research to explore this has been done in social work so far. The existing studies give the impression that, particularly when social work was being established at the beginning of the twentieth century, social workers and researchers took great pains to make knowledge from other nation-state contexts accessible in their own countries (Hegar 2008; Schüler 2004; Konrad 2009). Treptow and Walther (2010) surmise that the exchange across national borders mainly has to do with the fact that the crises of nineteenth-century social life in the developing industrial nations of Europe and North America have to be read as transnational crises. Their thesis is that these parallel developments of the industrialised states in Europe and America led to ideas and theories being received and applied cross-nationally. An important part was played by strong international social movements which arose in reaction to these social inequalities and ensured a positive reception for their ideas and theories across national borders. The international workers' movement, the women's movement, and the Red Cross movement can be cited as examples (Treptow 2004).

So although social work has become more aware of its transnational history in recent years, the existing literature does not usually clarify the significance of the nation-state for this exchange. Lorenz (2006) is one of the few to emphasise the importance of the nation-state for the history of social work in this context. He shows that schools and the welfare state are the central institutions through which the traditional forms of collectivisation (such as family and communities) are extended to the nation-state as a whole: "The nation constitutes its identity through these educational efforts, through not leaving the socialisation of its young to chance" (ibid.: 32). Social education is thus an essential strategy for ensuring that the population sees itself as part of an "imagined community" (Anderson 1983). The increasing awareness of transnational and global phenomena reveals the cracks in this imagining. This gives rise to new questions for social work: what function does social work have in the creation and maintenance of this central imagining of modernity? How has social work positioned itself in relation to this imagined national unity? What role do transnational practices of knowledge play?

## THE EXAMPLE OF THE SETTLEMENT MOVEMENT

These questions will now be analysed using the example of the settlement movement at the beginning of the twentieth century. The settlement movement is considered one of the main roots of professional social work in Great Britain and North America, as well as in Germany (Müller 1982; Sachße 1986; Wendt 2008). The starting point for this movement was social segregation, which was becoming visible in urban areas and was seen as increasingly problematic. Since the mid-nineteenth century, the compartmentalisation of the various population groups in the large cities of the industrialised western nation-states had increasingly come to be seen as a scandal. Schreiber (1904: 1) describes this sudden focus on and criticism of the social divide somewhat sarcastically:

> Between the seventies and eighties of the old century, London was gripped by 'slum fever'. This was not a malignant disease which spread from the overpopulated, dirty streets of the East, the so-called 'slums', into the capital city, but rather a sudden, feverish interest on the part of the educated in getting to know the long-ignored dens of poverty, as if they were a completely new discovery, rather than something long in existence, which had evolved gradually, over a period of decades, bit by bit.

This "slum fever" developed into criticism of a form of social work which limited itself to seeing the poor only as people in need of help. Instead, for parts of the bourgeoisie a conviction arose that it was necessary to move closer to the poor and the workers. This led to the idea of establishing settlements of so-called "educated" people (Picht 1913) in these districts, to come into contact with the workers and the poor as "neighbours" and to get to understand them better, to offer them educational opportunities, and thus to counteract the social divide. One of the founding declarations of the settlement movement—a lecture by Canon Samuel Barnett[5] delivered to a group of young men at St. John's College in Oxford in 1883—clearly shows this linking of social criticism and social work, typical of the settlement movement:

> Many have been the schemes of reform I have known, but, out of eleven years' experience, I would say that none touches the root of the evil which does not bring helper and helped into friendly relations. ( . . . ) Not until the habits of the rich are changed, and they are again content to breathe the same air and walk the same streets as the poor, will East London be 'saved'. Meantime a Settlement of University men will do a little to remove the inequalities of life, as the settlers share their best with the poor and learn through feeling how they live. (Barnett and Barnett 1915: 104–5)

Numerous settlement houses were subsequently established on the model of Toynbee Hall, not only in England, but also in the U.S. (Davis 1967). There in particular, the settlement movement evolved, quantitatively and qualitatively, into a constitutive factor for social work. Historic research has concentrated on the successful settlements in Boston, New York, and in particular Chicago, where the most famous settlement, Hull House, was founded by Jane Addams and Ellen Gates Star (Carson 1990).

As a rule, the transnational development[6] of the settlement movement is emphasised in this context. Still, there has been no precise historical analysis of the significance of this transnational knowledge production. Generally, the path of the settlement movement is traced from its founding in England, via its vigorous expansion in the U.S., to its spread into nearly all the industrial nations of North America and Europe.[7] As to the dissemination of ideas, the settlement movement resembles other international social movements and organisations at the time. However, some social movements, such as the international women's movement, were more aware of the fact that the international exchange of knowledge involves amendments, struggles, and negotiations about certain issues. A good example of this kind of transformation is the research on imperialism in international's women organisations conducted by Rupp (1996), and how it was challenged by women of the so-called Third World. To date, however, there exist no analyses of the transformations of the settlement idea and the importance of the nation-state context. This is all the more astonishing given that the social work discussion of the time highlighted the differences between settlements in the respective nation-states.

Thus for example Jane Addams speaks of "social settlements," in contrast to the English settlement movement, in order to emphasise the reform-oriented position of the American settlement movement (Addams 1892). Coit (1892), who was of vital importance for the development of the settlements in New York, also criticises the English settlements for not focusing on the "social reconstruction" of society. The differences between the nation-states were also highlighted from a sociological point of view. In his discussion of the basic functions of the settlements, Mead (1907–8: 108–9) argues:

> It is an interesting fact that settlements have flourished only where there has been a real democracy. Neither France, with its layers of society, its social castes, nor Germany, with its fundamental assumption that the control of society must take place from above through highly trained bureaus, have offered favorable soil for the growth of settlements. In France it is mutually impossible for men in different social groups to domesticate in other groups. In Germany nobody out of his own immediate milieu undertaking to enter into relations with others is at ease unless he has on a uniform indicating by what right he seeks information, gives advice, or renders assistance.

These examples show the rarely questioned assumption that differences emerge along national boundaries. In particular, Mead's reasoning about the dissemination of the settlement idea operates with an unquestioned assumption concerning notions of the nation, democracy, and cultural characteristics.

However, the aim of these quotes is not to reveal the questionable conjecture that national contexts determine the particular type of settlement work within a nation-state. Instead, they are intended to elucidate the fact that a *comparative perspective* on the settlements presupposes the nation-state as an independent, explanatory variable. As shown earlier, however, the nation-state is not a given, but a modern institution which is periodically reproduced. Thus, an examination of the transnational exchange of knowledge (both in the settlement movement and in social work) must consider two questions: not just how does the nation-state influence the knowledge production of the settlement movement, but also, conversely, to what extent does the knowledge production of the settlement movement contribute to the production of the nation-state?

The following analysis takes the latter question as its main starting point and reveals how various ideas concerning the settlement work of different (national) origin influenced the understanding of settlements in Germany and how these ideas became intertwined and intermingled in the imagined German national context.

## LETTERS FROM AMERICAN SETTLEMENTS

To this end, we delve into a series of letters about the American settlements sent to Germany by Alix Westerkamp during her stay in Chicago between November 1913 and May 1914, only months before the outbreak of World War I. These letters were printed in twelve episodes, between 1917 and 1919, in the journal *Akademisch-Soziale Monatsschrift* (Academic Social Monthly) and were written at a time when the settlement movement was about to reach the peak of its significance: the most important ideas had already been developed and the well-known social settlements were already widely recognized in the developing field of social work and social welfare. These settlements, such as Hull House, Chicago Commons, and Toynbee Hall, were seen as prototypes for the establishment of settlement houses in other large cities of the industrialised world. Therefore, production of knowledge concerning settlement work as expressed in these kinds of letters, publications, and talks used to be very common. However, the particular significance of these letters results from the relationship between the author of the letters, the Chicago Commons, and its founder Graham Taylor.

## CONTEXTUAL BACKGROUND OF THE LETTERS FROM AMERICAN SETTLEMENTS

Alix Westerkamp had a lasting but for the most part overlooked influence on the settlement movement in Germany and on work in the most prominent settlement, the Soziale Arbeitsgemeinschaft Berlin-Ost (SAG Berlin-Ost, East Berlin Social Working Group). Unlike the founder of the SAG Berlin-Ost, Friedrich Siegmund-Schultze, Westerkamp's influence on settlement work in Berlin, and that of the other collaborators, has hardly been researched to date. Thanks to the prominent role of Friedrich Siegmund-Schultze, the focus so far has been on the influence of the English settlements on the SAG Berlin-Ost (Scherer 2004; Lindner 1997). As a Protestant minister he had close connections with Protestant churches in England and was co-founder of the "*Church Committee for friendly relations between Great Britain and Germany*" (Siegmund-Schultze 1990: 47). He was strongly influenced by a visit in 1908, which took him to the poorest parts of East London. There he encountered the work being done in the first settlement in Great Britain, Toynbee Hall, founded in 1884 by Henrietta and Samuel Barnett.

Rarely mentioned, however, is the influence of the American settlements on Germany. For example, Friedrich Siegmund-Schultze visited American settlements such as Hull House for the first time in 1911 (Siegmund-Schultze 1990). Even more important was Alix Westerkamp's visit to the Chicago Commons. These experiences obviously influenced her decision to become part of the Soziale Arbeitsgemeinschaft, yet her involvement had begun much earlier and coincided with the establishment of the Soziale Arbeitsgemeinschaft in East Berlin. As the first woman to obtain a doctorate in law in Germany (Röwekamp 2005), she initially headed (from 1907) the Rechtschutzstelle für Frauen (women's legal protection centre) in Frankfurt am Main, before moving to Berlin in 1911 and taking charge of the Deutsche Zentrale für Jugendfürsorge (DZfJ, German centre for youth care). This was the context for her first contact with Siegmund-Schultze in the summer of 1911. When the latter was looking for a place to establish the SAG, he turned to Westerkamp.[8] Based on her previous experience in the context of the Berlin Jugendgerichtshilfe (juvenile court assistance), she advised him to take the area around the "Schlesischer Bahnhof" as a starting point. This area was considered the home of many labourers who were alienated from the church but were involved in the communist, socialist, and social democratic parties of the time. The SAG Berlin-Ost was in fact founded in this area that same year, at Friedensstrasse 60.

Westerkamp managed the DZfJ for two years before leaving on her study trip to Chicago, where she spent several months becoming acquainted with settlement work in the Chicago Commons. Even though she did not mention in her letters why she opted for the Chicago Commons rather than for the far better known Hull House of Jane Addams, two explanations are possible: First, its founder and first director, Graham Taylor, was a Protestant clergyman, just as was Friedrich Siegmund-Schultze. Both were engaged in the international peace movement and they probably knew each other from Friedrich Siegmund-Schultze's visit in 1911. Second, this settlement house was situated in an area where many German immigrants used to live. As Alix Westerkamp intended to volunteer as a settlement worker, the Chicago Commons was a perfect place to make use of her language abilities and her aspiration to contribute to settlement work. After her return from the U.S., she became a close collaborator of Siegmund-Schultze and edited the *Akademisch-Soziale Monatsschrift* with him from 1917 to 1924 (Röwekamp 2005).

The Chicago Commons was founded in 1894 by Graham Taylor, who "was one of the first to introduce sociology or social ethics into the curriculum of a theological school" (Davis 1967: 13). While this settlement house had a religious background, its main emphasis lay on social reform and democratic development. Because of this combination of religious and societal impetus, the Chicago Commons was an often-referred-to example, especially in large cities such as Toronto, where the churches used to play an important role (Fraser 1988; James 1997). This characteristic also made it interesting for the German settlement movement, especially for the Soziale Arbeitsgemeinschaft Berlin-Ost with its Protestant background. In fact, German class conflict bore greater resemblance to the social circumstances in the UK, but the focus on social reform and democracy was of great interest to German settlement workers, who found themselves in a highly unstable political and societal context at the end of World War I.

## THE LETTERS

An overview of the range of themes covered by Alix Westerkamp in her nineteen letters will clarify the structure and the themes under discussion. She wrote her letters mainly in the Chicago Commons, which was—as she says—the oldest and biggest settlement in Chicago, after Hull House. She writes about Graham Taylor with "endless" admiration (Westerkamp 1917–19, II: 49),[9] but is initially unable to establish a close relationship with him.

The dominant motif of the letters becomes clear in the first sentences of her first letter on 16 November 1913: "I'd rather tell you about where and how I'm living next time. I'm still too new here. But I've already seen a great deal of Young America. Young America! What is it? It's Young Italy, Young Poland, Young Hungary, Young Bohemia, Young Slovenia and Slovania, Young Norway and Sweden, Young England, Scotland and Ireland, Young France, Young Germany, and—last but not least—a young Jewry. But all of them are becoming a young, vigorous America." This America—above all its political culture and the socio-political challenges it faces—continues to preoccupy Westerkamp in subsequent letters. She makes comparisons with Germany mainly to emphasise the otherness of life in the U.S. For example, she writes in the first letter: "I get the impression that the young people here are taller and stronger than in the old world. It's as if they have more room to grow, and therefore flourish like free-standing trees. In Germany a certain lack of physical agility is often seen as naturally connected with Jewishness. Here the young Jews play the sport of Young America from an early age, and they become just as sinewy and tall and straight as the others" (ibid. I: 21).

Her letters read like a sort of autoethnography. She describes her struggle with the adverse conditions in Chicago (wind, dust, dirt, and noise), her own foreignness, of which she is particularly conscious on such occasions as Christmas and Easter, and finally, in the last letters, her illness ("a simple grip"), which confines her to bed for several weeks and takes her to a sanatorium 60 km west of Chicago. The settlement work itself is also described wholly from a subjective point of view. Westerkamp does not write about something she is observing, but describes how she herself experiences the settlement work, how she becomes acquainted with American "living conditions" during her "investigations" in Chicago, how she makes contact with German families, how she rescues a family from death by suffocation, how disconcerting she finds the American Christmas celebration with its songs, whose lyrics (*Oh tree of fir*) are wrongly assumed to be English originals, the red Christmas decorations, which remind her not of Christmas but of a socialist rally, etc. The manner in which she proceeds is characteristic of the attitude of the settlement workers: by means of a more participant than observing attitude they try to understand and describe social worlds from the inside out (Wietschorke 2006), whether it be the local Berlin neighbourhood, work in a factory, or settlement work in another country.

It is not until 2 December 1913, in the third published letter, that she discusses the settlement work in the Chicago Commons in more detail. As at the beginning of the first letter, she starts by highlighting a difference between Germany and America: "In Germany there is only very little which is similar; our problems are quite different to those of the United States. Here the problem of nationalities is a defining one for almost all social work." In the entrance hall to the Chicago Commons she is impressed by a quotation from Homer: "He was a friend to man and he lived by the side of the road."[10] This quotation, she concludes, is the real "leitmotif of the settlements." This short motif alludes to the metaphor of the "neighbour" which is central for the settlement movement (Irving, Parsons, and Bellamy 1995). The settlement workers settle where they can meet their fellow humans, where they can immerse themselves in their everyday life and culture, and where they can offer help to those who seek it. Westerkamp sees this goal of settlement work as closely connected to the task of "turning the immigrants into useful 'American citizens'" (Westerkamp 1917–19, I: 28).

This leitmotif of settlement work reveals strong parallels to an experience which she places in a broader context. That which preoccupies Westerkamp almost more than the actual settlement work is the political and social culture of America. On 7 January 1914 she begins one of her most forceful letters on the subject with the following words: "Your Christmas letter is there, with its 'Christmas sermon'. Its 'text' inspired what has perhaps been my greatest and most wonderful experience here in the United States" (ibid. IV: 120). She is referring to a letter from Germany whose author is unnamed, and as she later adds in a footnote, the text she is alluding to comes from "A Christmas Carol" by Charles Dickens: "But I am sure I have always thought of Christmas time . . . as a good time: a kind, forgiving, charitable, pleasant time: the only time I know of, in the long calendar of the year, when men and women seem by one consent to open their shut-up hearts freely, and to think of people below them as if they really were fellow-passengers to the grave, and not another race of creatures bound on other journeys." She describes the experience inspired by the text in contrast with her everyday life in Germany: "In Germany, the class differences constantly assert themselves everywhere. Anyone who has any feeling for this at all senses them as a physical pressure. Never, in all the joyless manifestations of our public life, which are to be addressed as consequences of class differences, have I been able to rid myself of the feeling: mea maxima culpa" (ibid. IV: 120).

In contrast, in her eyes American life is infused with the conviction that people are in principle equal and have equal rights:

> It is unbelievably different to Germany—life in the street, in the tram, in the train, in assemblies, in public buildings. The people are, to quote your Christmas sermon, *'fellow passengers'*, not just at Christmas, but all year round. The wonderful words of the Declaration of Independence, *'that all men are created equal'*—they're not literally fulfilled, just as they're not intended to be understood literally, but they're *at least somewhat of a reality here*. The differences are there—differences in wealth, in education, in social position, and many others, just like in our country, but in everyday life those who are at a disadvantage

are not constantly reminded of this—it is not cudgelled into them, as it were. (ibid. IV: 120f., italicised quotes in English in the original text)

What is interesting in this quote is not only the fabulous creolisation of the language in itself (which includes English and English-influenced phrases), but the idea which Westerkamp is expressing thereby. She brings her different experiences in Germany and the U.S. together, but they refuse to merge and create a unity. Westerkamp is caught in a process of transition which puts her in a state of personal tension, for in spite of her euphoric description of everyday life in America she notes two lines later: "Never have I been more passionately German, never have I felt more consciously that one is rooted with one's innermost values in the soil of one's native land" (ibid.).

This general, fairly abstract insight is illustrated in the same letter with an example. First she describes a "political scandal" which preoccupied Chicago around the end of 1913 and the beginning of 1914. This occurred in the "Board of Education," to which Ella Flagg-Young was, surprisingly, not re-elected as chairwoman, although she—as Westerkamp presumes—[must] have achieved wonderful things" (ibid. IV: 122). Instead, her former assistant, "quite a good politician, but not an educator" (ibid.), became chairman on the basis of a "terrible intrigue" (ibid.). "A storm of indignation raged through Chicago" (ibid.), and mass meetings were held, demanding that politics should cease to influence the administration. The "people's will" ("des Volkes Wille") triumphed in the end, and Ella Flagg-Young became chairwoman again. Westerkamp draws the conclusion that she had already hinted at earlier: "One learns an incredible amount from such an event. It's also quite healthy for someone who has perhaps been too burdened by Germany's air to see that too, perfection is still an unattained goal. One thing, however, was clear from the beginning: that Chicago would find a way out of this difficulty. The Americans have a tremendous energy for higher development in their constitutional life" (ibid.). For her, the United States is not the ideal model because it differs with respect to the fundamental issue of the settlement movement, the segregation into rich and poor. Instead, it is distinguished by a sort of basic political and social structure in which the "history of a people (*Volk*) with such a decisive talent for politics" (ibid. V: 154) manifests itself. Westerkamp, in her system of motifs, closely links this basic political-social structure to the work in the settlements. The motifs of the "fellow passenger" and the "friend to man" produce the picture of an *elective affinity* between the strategies of the settlement workers and the already existing basic political-social structure.

Westerkamp gives further examples of this basic message about the political culture in subsequent letters. In the following three striking aspects may be identified. On 28 January 1914 she recounts a typical "American destiny" (ibid. VI: 184), using this case to illustrate the difference between the political landscapes in the two countries. During one of her late-evening "investigations" she has been accompanied by a co-worker from the Chicago

Commons. She has always considered this man to be of a "scholarly nature" and was therefore all the more astonished when it transpired that he came from a steel-working family. Full of admiration, she recounts his story: how his father died of tuberculosis, his mother encouraged him to see his fate as "not unchangeable," and he earned money as a steelworker until he saved enough to be able to go to university. Even in Germany, such a career is not impossible, Westerkamp concedes. She wonders, however, why such people are almost all to be found among the ranks of the Social Democrats in Germany, while this is not the case in the U.S. (ibid. VI: 185).

One letter later, on the topic of the political situation of women, she reports enthusiastically on the introduction of women's suffrage and on the "political education" being provided "by women for women" (ibid. VI: 186). Political issues are "discussed with a seriousness, with a thoroughness and an interest . . . which astonish me" (ibid.), and not only among women in fashionable clubs, but also among the "simplest and poorest women, whom we are accustomed to classify as 'washerwomen and cleaning ladies'" (ibid.).

Finally, on 11 February, she discusses the national celebrations on the birthdays of Abraham Lincoln (12 February 1809) and George Washington (22 February 1732). She compares these with the "jubilee of our emperor" (ibid. VIII: 54) from the previous year, when she walked along Unter den Linden—a central boulevard of Berlin—and heard a voice from the festive crowd saying: "'Well, tout Berlin[11] is here.' This 'tout Berlin' made me flinch. Where were the people from the North and the East, from Neukölln and Lichtenberg,[12] where were 'the people' ('das Volk')? Who remembered that countless people ( . . . ) had no part, not the even the tiniest part in their emperor's jubilee? Can you call that a *national* holiday?" (ibid., emphasis in original). In contrast, the "national holidays" in the U.S. live up to their name, according to Westerkamp. She cites two assemblies as evidence of this: for one, a meeting of the "Mother's Club," in which the previously mentioned "washerwomen and cleaning ladies" come together, and from whose midst "the spontaneous wish [arose] for their celebration to begin with a lecture about George Washington" (ibid.). Secondly, a "negro gathering" (ibid. VIII: 56), which makes it clear to her that the "negro question" has not yet been solved, but that the blacks are nonetheless recognised by the white population as having equal rights—in complete contrast to Germany, where anti-Semitism illustrates the systematic disadvantaging of certain population groups (ibid.).

Her experiences with American political life also change her perspective on the work in the settlement. One manifestation of this is the way she reports on this work. For example, the second and third compilations of letters (10, 17, 24, and 31 December) still focus on the characteristic of cultural diversity, and on the major challenge faced by the Chicago Commons because of its location in a district where the ethnic and social composition is constantly changing. After the foregoing quoted letters on everyday political-social life in January, in the middle of February (14 and 19 February 1914) she returns to the description of the actual work in the settlement but now she places more emphasis on the significance of the settlement's political attitude and work. For example, she describes her experiences with a group of Italian men during a game evening in the auditorium: "You should see these young Romans around the table, flashing eyes, burning cheeks, and unconsciously, fantastically grand, picturesque gestures. And for all their temperament and passion a certain respect for parliamentary form which seems to become second nature to anyone who grows up here" (ibid. IX: 92). It is not entirely by chance that the indexical "here" in the second sentence is ambiguous: does it refer to the settlement, Chicago, or the U.S.?

This parliamentary attitude seems, for her, to infuse all aspects of life in this settlement. She writes almost emotionally about a daily routine, the "Vesper." For her this meeting after dinner, devoted to the discussion of a current event from the city or state, from social work or personal life, is like an "hour of consecration for the whole day" (ibid. X: 122). The description of the meetings and the name remind one of a religious ceremony with a profane or rather socio-political content. On one of these evenings the topic is a miners' strike which kept the U.S. on tenterhooks in 1913 and 1914. She is impressed both by the events surrounding this strike, and by Graham Taylor's knowledge of the political situation relating to this conflict. Her summary includes a sarcastic dig at Germany: "And as with the national holidays, I can't help thinking again here: how could it be otherwise? . . . In the end, every country has the social democracy it deserves" (ibid. X: 123).

The last letters of Westerkamp display a deeper immersion into the everyday life of Chicago and an adoption of the mythology of the American dream (in particular, the equality of opportunity and the ability to solve existing problems). Therefore, her experiences in the U.S. deepen her criticism of the German situation. The extent to which this affects her personally becomes clear in the last letter, before she becomes ill for several months. On 25 February 1914, on the occasion of Washington's birthday, she took part in a celebration dedicated to the new arrivals in the city and the country. Deeply moved, she quotes extensively from the speech given by a representative of the government, who emphasised the significance of every individual and of the people (*Volk*) as a whole for the development of the country. She contrasts this with her evening reading of a newspaper which has a "foreign part" once a week: "With greedy eyes I looked for 'Germany'. I had such a longing to read something which would make my heart beat faster, and I found. . . . the Zabern affair. A chill seized me. I thought it was a mental chill. But since then I've been ill" (ibid. X: 126). Of course this is just a coincidence. And yet the contrast could scarcely be more extreme. Here the United States, which presents itself to Westerkamp as a democratic country, there Germany, where the military inflicts arbitrary force on the populace in Alsace (in this case Zabern/Saverne); here a country which—in Westerkamp's view—welcomes all people equally, there a country rife with racist, nationalist, and class-specific resentments.

## CONCLUSIONS

The analysis of Alix Westerkamp's letters is significant for the question of transnational knowledge production in social work in three respects. First, it provides concrete information about the settlement movement and its transnational knowledge production and shows how these ideas travelled through space and time, and how they were transformed and translated in other contexts. Second, it reveals the ambivalent meaning of boundary objects such as the nation and the people (*Volk*) in these practices of trans-nationalising knowledge. Third and finally, such an analysis gives rise to new perspectives on the question of how transnational practices—and the correspondence between the U.S. and Germany undoubtedly counts as one of these—relate to methodological nationalism in social work.

1. Alix Westerkamp describes *settlement work* and the *settlement movement* not as a method for solving particular social problems, but as a movement which sees itself as embedded in a general political development, which is concerned with the pursuit of social and political goals. She there-fore only describes the settlement work in the Chicago Commons in a small part of her letters, and instead concentrates in large part on the political and social developments in Chicago and the U.S. She regards the settlement movement as a crucial means of advancing reforms, especially at a national level. Even where she deals with the subject of the political-social setting of Chicago by recounting the events after Ella Flagg-Young was voted out of her position as chair of the Board of Education, she eventually also refers to the socio-political culture in the U.S. in its entirety. Westerkamp sketches a picture of a settlement movement which pursues, almost as a matter of course, the goal of instigating political-social reform in a particular nation-state context, the U.S. in this case. In sum, her letters describe a reform movement which is situated in a neighbourhood but is ultimately concerned with the *nation*.

With terms such as the nation or the people (das Volk) she refers to a decisive connecting piece of the settlement movement, one which has not been adequately explored. The idea of establishing settlements in the poor areas of large cities developed in a discursive field in which authors from very different ideological backgrounds—for example, Friedrich Engels (German socialist), Léon Faucher (French liberal), William Cooke Taylor (Irish Whig)— criticised the fact that the "rich abandoned their responsibil-ity for morality and order among the working classes" (Dennis 1980: 315). The emergence of "two nations," as Benjamin Disraeli, the romantic writer and conservative prime minister, put it in 1845, was considered a serious threat to the nation-state (in this case, the United Kingdom). The metaphor of the two nations was influential for the settlement movement but has been interpreted in very different ways in different contexts.

Samuel Barnett, for example, viewed this disparity as a result of spatial segregation and a lack of education and knowledge. With reference to the English settlement movement, Allen F. Davis points out: "[It] was part of the larger Romantic revolt against the vulgarization of society, and its ultimate goal was the spiritual reawakening of the whole man—and not just the labourer, but the university man also" (Davis 1967: 7). Barnett thus considered the divided nation to be a crisis of the nation in the sense of an *educated community*. In other words, education and communication promoted by spatial permeation were the cure that was envisaged for the nation.

Jane Addams (1899) also took up the question of the two nations in her article "A Function of the Social Settlement." She argues in opposition to Disraeli's diagnosis: "We do not like to acknowledge that Americans are divided into 'two nations,' as her prime minister once admitted of England. ( . . . ) Our democracy is still our most precious possession, and we do well to resent any inroads upon it, even although they may be made in the name of philanthropy" (ibid.: 33). Her reference to the democratic system in the U.S. elucidates her conception of the nation: it is above all a *political community*. She does not deny the analysis of social inequality within the U.S. but she obviously believes in the idea of a political way of tackling these challenges. Her favoured strategy resembles Barnett's vision of a settlement only at first glance: She is also persuaded that "the most pressing problem of modern life is that of a reconstruction and a reorganization of the knowledge which we possess" (ibid.: 34). But reorganisation of knowledge means not only sharing the knowledge with the poor—for example, through education. With reference to pragmatic academics such as John Dewey, she demands first and foremost the application of social science knowledge to the benefit of the poor, especially in areas where it is most needed. In sum, social settlements are a way of building a nation as a *knowledgeable community*.

Because of the strong antagonism between the bourgeoisie and the working class, the question of the nation and the nation-state was an even more important issue within the German settlement movement than elsewhere. Friedrich Siegmund-Schultze takes up the metaphor of Disraeli in an unpublished manuscript with the title "Two people" (*Zwei Völker*) (EZA 626/I 6: 2). He describes one people as the old one "that lives in remembrance of the history of its ancestors, having grown up in victorious wars; . . . proud of its strength, at the same time in possession of the entire national tradition;" the other people, the new one, is considered to be "without national tradition, . . . raised . . . in the peaceful and international development of industry and technology, nowhere rooted in the soil, . . . thus viewing the world as its homeland." Although Siegmund-Schultze searches for a conciliatory position between these two peoples, in other publications he leaves no doubt about the deficiencies of this new people: "And after all one fact is undeniable: a dreadful mass disease is currently spreading through our nation. The hostility to God has become epidemic" (1990: 298). This quote illustrates the fact that Siegmund-Schultze regards the national division not only as a social issue but also as a moral one. Seen from this angle, settlements attempt to overcome the gap between the socialist-oriented and atheistic labourers, on the one hand, and the bourgeois church, on the other. In other words, he considers the sharp opposition of the social classes in Germany to be a crisis of the nation as a *moral community.*

Alix Westerkamp's letters from an American settlement were written at the intersection of these different conceptions of the nation and nation-state which emerged before and after the beginning of the settlement movement. Two conceptions of the nation dominate her reports. First of all, her passionate account of the feelings of guilt and depression in her thoughts about the class conflict in Germany reveals her view of the nation as a *moral community.* Her tendency to use religious metaphors also underlines this notion, which she shares with Siegmund-Schultze. Instead of dwelling on the problem of irreligiosity, however, she focuses decisively on the political culture of the U.S. and its ability to overcome not only the economic gap but also the religious, gender, and racial differences within the nation-state. The so-called "Vesper" in the Chicago Commons stands paradigmatically for her move toward a political overcoming of societal (i.e., religious, economical, gendered, etc.) disparities. This daily ceremony is a religiously based yet profane event in which the settlement movement manifests its aspiration to become the nucleus of a *political community.* This second view ultimately sublates (in the Hegelian sense) the previous conception, since Westerkamp considers a political approach to be suitable for overcoming, or at least lessening, the moral disparities within the nation.

2. The utilisation of the polymorphic notion of a nation and a people (*Volk*), which we have previously analysed, has implications for the question *concerning the ways in which knowledge is produced transnationally and the consequences thereof.* Westerkamp's letters can undoubtedly be taken as an important example of the way in which ideas and knowledge circulated across borders in early twentieth-century social work. Like Werner Picht (1913), for example, whose book *Toynbee Hall and the English Settlement Movement* was an important contribution to the spread of this idea in Germany, she too chooses the route of long-term observing participation. She condenses these personal and physically very strenuous experiences into letters, which are then published in the *Akademisch-Soziale Monatsschrift*, mainly for the benefit of those with a professional interest in the subject. Although she uses such categories as 'people' (*Volk*) and 'nation' fairly sparingly, they do nonetheless play a central role as frames of reference. Though she does not state this explicitly, Westerkamp seems to perceive a sort of *elective affinity* between the U.S. and the settlement movement. The principles of the settlement are reflected, in her view, in a particular U.S. political-social culture, and vice versa. The impression emerges that this is the place where the idea of the settlement movement

can have its full effect. One could borrow Westerkamp's quip and say: just as every country has the social democracy it deserves, so does every country have its corresponding settlement movement.

Such constructions have interesting implications for the circulation of knowledge and ideas. Tying settlement work to a specific national context in this way means that it cannot simply be imitated and transferred as a strategy. Contemporaries and readers of the *Akademisch-Soziale Monatsschrift* will probably be wondering what conclusions can be drawn from Westerkamp's experiences for settlement work in Germany. She herself gives no direct answer to this. By constructing an elective affinity, however, she creates a dilemma for her readers: they are presented with an interesting 'model,' which nevertheless does not seem usable, or at least not in this form. These unique experiences also seem to create a dilemma for Westerkamp herself. The apparently enormous discrepancies between the U.S. and Germany frustrate her intensely. The 'mental' chill which seizes her is symptomatic of her feelings of resignation and hopelessness. On the one hand she is enthusiastic about the idea of settlement work and about the political-social culture in the U.S. On the other hand, this brings home to her how much the situation in Germany oppresses her—although or particularly because she feels more passionately German than ever before.

The significance of the frame of reference of a nationally influenced political-social culture draws attention to an elementary mechanism of transnational knowledge production. With terms like people (*Volk*) and nation, Westerkamp chooses terms which are important 'anchor points' for both the readers of her letters in Germany and for the settlement movement. Talking about the nation and the *Volk* is, for Westerkamp, a sort of *boundary object*, with which she can connect her experiences in the U.S. with her readers' horizon of experience. In the sociology of scientific knowledge, the significance of such boundary objects has long been acknowledged:

> Boundary objects are both plastic enough to adapt to local needs and constraints of several parties employing them, yet robust enough to maintain a common identity across sites. They are weakly structured in common use, and become strongly structured in individual-site use. They may be abstract or concrete. They have different meanings in different social worlds but their structure is common enough to more than one world to make them recognisable means of translation. The creation and management of boundary objects is a key in developing and maintaining coherence across intersecting social worlds. (Star and Griesemer 1989: 393)

The analysis of Westerkamp's letters shows that she avoids using terms such as *Volk* and nation. She does not make it too easy for her readers. With terms such as American life, America, American citizen; with comparisons (to Germany) and with strategically placed narrative she emphasises the individuality of the U.S. and—through the comparison with Germany—that of nations and national developments in general. And yet boundary objects such as nation or *Volk* reveal a paradox. They make it possible for different actors from different social contexts to refer to these concepts. But at the same time they are boundary objects which entail a construction of uniqueness. For the settlement movement, such terms are even able to create a common identity, as shown by Lies Benzler's (1926) account of the second congress of the international settlement movement in Paris. She quotes the chairman of the Federation of British Settlements: "He emphasised the paradoxical aspect of an international settlement conference. Every settlement, he said, began with a national goal: it sought to help its own people (*Volk*) to achieve unity. Thus every country, he continued, had its own particular problems and challenges. But out of the protest against evil in each individual people (*Volk*), a goal for the whole of humanity arose. In the settlement movement, he argued, sincere 'nationalism' ended in 'internationalism'" (Benzler 1926: 46). By referring to a nation as a quasi-natural frame of reference, all the members of the settlement movement reassure each other of their commonality. The quote also shows the self-evident quality of the nation as an almost natural organisation of the social world at the time, even in a social movement that is, to a great extent, involved in the international peace movement (for example, Jane Addams, Friedrich Siegmund-Schultze). At the same time, however, this common point of reference generates a marked difference between the actors, which can only be overcome through the construction of a paradox, with nationalism ultimately merging into internationalism—though why this should be so remains unanswered.

3. This result, finally, throws new light on the question of how a *methodological nationalism* has been able to arise in social work. Westerkamp's letters about the "American settlements" are evidence of a transnational production of knowledge. But in this knowledge production, the boundary objects nation and people (*Volk*) acquire a life of their own: they reinforce the impression of the otherness and uniqueness of the settlement work which Westerkamp is observing. In other words, Westerkamp's transnational practice[13] ultimately leads to a reinforcement of the nation-state frame of reference, even if this was probably not her intention. The example shows, however, that a transnational production of knowledge does not necessarily lead to a reduction in national differences. On the contrary, nationalisms can actually be intensified by certain practices of comparison, and by the establishment of boundary objects that not only connect different actors but also divide them by emphasising the particular characteristics of certain actors such as nations.

In the case of the settlement movement, this paradoxical logic of the term 'nation' is intensified through its ideological framework. Not only by seeking to support the poor or to overcome the segregation of the poor and the rich within large cities, but also by reconstructing and reforming the nation and the nation-state, the settlement movement regards the solution of social problems to be a national endeavour. Many settlement workers were skeptical about the focus of professionalised social work on individual cases and favoured the idea that all the societal actors should participate in the campaign against social divisions within the nation-state. Settlement houses were seen as both the pivotal core of this reform and as an anchor for the different actors within the nation-state. Although settlement workers did not promote the methodological nationalism of social work, they nonetheless were furthering a kind of *progressive and reformative nationalism* during this period.

## NOTES

1. In this context, methodological nationalism has to be distinguished from normative nationalism, which is a political premise that denotes the right of nations and nation-states to self-determination. Still, the two perspectives are interlinked: the unquestioned premise of the social sciences, according to which the confines of the nation-state represent the quasi-natural confines of social life, refers back to the everyday assumptions of political and everyday actors.
2. This sharp and comprehensive criticism of the social sciences did not remain unchallenged (Chernilo 2006). Particularly questioned was the diagnosis that the classical grand theories would follow a methodological nationalism. I will not discuss this criticism in more detail because it is not relevant to the following argument.
3. New institutionalism is a theoretical reference point for research, especially in the field of organisational studies. This approach reflects the societal embeddedness of organisations and the legitimacy organisations gain by adopting structures and practices that could be found in the environments of these organisations (which are called organisational fields). In particular, Meyer (2009) with his world polity analyses focuses on macro-sociological phenomena and the global diffusion of institutions.
4. Historical research on social work, especially research focusing on the transnational production of knowledge, faces the very important problem that the confines of social work are anything but determined or defined. Social work is not only differently understood in various time periods, but also in different social and cultural contexts. The research I am dealing with in this study is mainly related to what is called 'social work' in North America, the United Kingdom, and parts of Europe.
5. Samuel and Henrietta Barnett established the first settlement house, Toynbee Hall, in 1884. The name derives from Arnold Toynbee, an English economic historian who moved to Whitechapel, East London, in order to aid in improving the living conditions there. He died in 1883.
6. This development is considered transnational in so far as the transfer of ideas across national boundaries conveys a process of translation of these ideas into a new social and national context. This translation implies a revelation, reflection, and reconfirmation or modification of those nation-state institutions involved in this process (for example, language, territory, culture, and law). The goal of this definition is not to get a grasp of a certain scope, but a certain kind of phenomena.
7. Only a few settlements were founded in Asian cities such as Hong Kong and Manila.
8. His first intention was to start settlement work in an infamous Berlin neighbourhood called the Scheuenviertel. But the partial demolition of this district in 1907 and Siegmund-Schultze's aim of getting in contact with the "Berlin's healthy and hardy labour force" (Lindner 1997: 83) led to a reorientation.

9. The first six episodes were published in 1917, episodes 7 to 11 in 1918, and the last episode in 1919.
10. This Homerian motif was very popular at the time in Canada and the U.S., particularly because of a poem by Sam Walter Foss. While Alix Westerkamp does not mention this context, it is likely that Graham Taylor chose the Homer quotation in light of the popularity of this poem. The second stanza of the poem makes it clear that there are obvious parallels to the settlement idea: "Let me live in a house by the side of the road/ Where the race of men go by;/ The men who are good and the men who are bad,/ As good and as bad as I./ I would not sit in the scorner's seat/ Or hurl the cynic's ban;/ Let me live in a house by the side of the road/ And be a friend to man" (Foss 1897: 11).
11. Westerkamp quotes this French expression for "all of Berlin" literally, and in this way also indicates the bourgeois background of the narrator, since practicing French was fashionable in German bourgeoisie at the time.
12. Neukölln and Lichtenberg used to be independent, highly industrialised and congested cities in the Berlin area.
13. This is taken to mean the totality of the transnational practices of Alix Westerkamp and her target audience: from the participatory observation via the writing and reading of the letters to the publication, the renewed reading, quoting, and the analysis taking place here.

## BIBLIOGRAPHY

Addams, J. (1892) 'The Subjective Necessity for Social Settlements.' In *Philanthropy and Social Progress. Seven Essays*, edited by J. Addams, R. A. Woods, F. J. O. S. Huntington, F. H. Giddens, and B. Bosanquet, 1–26. New York: T. Y. Crowell.

Addams, J. (1899) 'A Function of the Social Settlement.' *The Annals of the American Academy of Political and Social Science*, 13(3): 33–55.

Anderson, B. (1983) *Imagined Communities: Reflections on the Origins and Spread of Nationalism*. London: Verso Ed.

Barnett, S. A., and H. Barnett (1915) *Practicable Socialism: New Series*. 3rd ed. London: Longmans.

Beck, U. (2000) *What Is Globalization?* Cambridge: Polity Press.

Benzler, L. (1926) 'Die 2. Internationale Settlement-Konferenz in Paris vom 1.-5. Juli 1926.' *Akademisch-Soziale Monatsschrift*, 10(3/4): 43–61.

Callon, M. (1980) 'Struggles and Negotiations to Define What Is Problematic and What Is Not: The Socio-logic of Translation.' In *The Social Process of Scientific Investigation*, edited by K. D. Knorr, R. Krohn, and R. Whitley, 197–221. Dordrecht [et al.]: Reidel.

Carson, M. J. (1990) *Settlement Folk: Social Thought and the American Settlement Movement 1885–1930*. Chicago: University of Chicago Press.

Chernilo, D. (2006) 'Social Theory's Methodological Nationalism: Myth and Reality.' *European Journal of Social Theory*, 9(1): 5–22.

Clifford, J. (1989) 'Notes on Travel and Theory.' *Inscriptions. Center for Cultural Studies journal* (5), http://www2.ucsc.edu/culturalstudies/PUBS/Inscriptions/vol_5/clifford.html (accessed: Oct. 27, 2011).

Coit, S. (1892) *Neighbourhood Guilds*. London: Swan Sonnenschein & Co.

Davis, A. F. (1967) *Spearheads for Reform: The Social Settlements and the Progressive Movement 1890–1914*. New York: Oxford University Press.

Dennis, R. J. (1980) 'More Thoughts on Victorian Cities.' *Area*, 12(4): 313–17.

Eickelpasch, R. (2002) 'Parteiliche Unparteilichkeit. Paradoxien in der Begründung einer kritischen Soziologie bei Pierre Bourdieu.' In *Theorie als Kampf? Zur politischen Soziologie Pierre Bourdieus*, edited by U. H. Bittlingmayer, R. Eickelpasch, J. Kastner, and C. Rademacher, 49–60. Opladen: Leske + Budrich.

EZA (Evangelisches Zentralarchiv/Evangelical Central Archive, Berlin) Serie 626: Friedrich Siegmund-Schultze.

Foss, S. W. (1897) *Dreams in Homespun*. Boston: Lothrop, Lee & Sheppard Co.

Fraser, B. J. (1988) *Social Uplifters: Presbyterian Progressives and the Social Gospel in Canada, 1875–1915*. Waterloo: Wilfrid Laurier Press.

Glick Schiller, N., L. Basch, and C. Blanc-Szanton, eds. (1992) *Towards a transnational perspective on migration: race, class, ethnicity, and nationalism reconsidered*. New York: New York Academy of Sciences.

Goldmann, L. (1973) *Der verborgene Gott. Studie über die tragische Weltanschauung in den Pensées Pascals und im Theater Racines* (Translation from French title: *Le dieu caché*, published by Gallimard (Paris) in 1955). Neuwied [et al.]: Luchterhand.

Haraway, D. J. (1991) *Simians, Cyborgs, and Women: The Reinvention of Nature*. London: Routledge.

Hasse, R., and G. Krücken (2005) *Neo-Institutionalismus*. 2., revised ed. Bielefeld: Transcript.

Hegar, R. L. (2008) 'Transatlantic Transfers in Social Work: Contributions of Three Pioneers.' *European Journal of Social Work*, 38(4): 716–33.

Irving, A., H. Parsons, and D. Bellamy (1995) *Neighbours: Three Social Settlements in Downtown Toronto*. Toronto: Canadian Scholars' Press.

James, C. L. (1997) *Gender, Class and Ethnicity in the Organization of Neighbourhood and Nation: The Role of Toronto's Settlement Houses in the Formation of the Canadian State, 1902 to 1914*. Toronto: University of Toronto.

Khagram, S., and P. Levitt (2008) 'Constructing Transnational Studies.' In *The Transnationals Studies Reader. Intersections and Innovations*, edited by S. Khagram and P. Levitt, 1–22, New York et al.: Routledge.

Köngeter, S. (2009) 'Der methodologische Nationalismus der Sozialen Arbeit in Deutschland.' *Zeitschrift für Sozialpädagogik*, 7(4): 340–59.

Konrad, F.-M. (2009) 'Ob das amerikanische Beispiel nachgeahmt werden kann . . . , läßt sich noch nicht abschließend beurteilen. Die Bedeutung des Ausland in den sozialpädagogischen Reformdebatten in Deutschland 1900–1933.' In *Innovation durch Grenzüberschreitung*, edited by F. Hamburger, 19–61. Bremen: Europ. Hochsch.-verl.

Latour, B., and S. Woolgar (1979) *Laboratory Life: The Social Construction of Scientific Facts*. Beverly Hills: Sage.

Lindner, R. (1997) 'Die Anfänge der Sozialen Arbeitsgemeinschaft Berlin-Ost.' In *"Wer in den Osten geht, geht in ein anderes Land"—Die Settlementbewegung in Berlin zwischen Kaiserreich und Weimarer Republik*, edited by R. Lindner, 82–94. Berlin: Akad.-Verl.

Lorenz, W. (2006) *Perspectives on European Social Work: From the Birth of the Nation State to the Impact of Globalisation*. Opladen: Budrich.

Mead, G. H. (1907–8) 'The Social Settlement: Its Basis and Function.' *University of Chicago Record*, 12: 108–10.

Meyer, J. W. (2009) *World Society: The Writings of John W. Meyer*, edited by G. Krücken and G. S. Drori. Oxford: Oxford University Press.

Müller, C. W. (1982) *Wie Helfen zum Beruf wurde. Eine Methodengeschichte der Sozialarbeit*. Weinheim: Beltz.

Picht, W. (1913) *Toynbee Hall und die englische Settlement-Bewegung: ein Beitrag zur Geschichte der sozialen Bewegung in England*. Tübingen: Mohr.

Pries, L. (2008) *Die Transnationalisierung der sozialen Welt: Sozialräume jenseits von Nationalgesellschaften*. Frankfurt a. M.: Suhrkamp.

Röwekamp, M., ed. (2005) *Juristinnen: Lexikon zu Leben und Werk*. Baden-Baden: Nomos-Verl.-Ges.

Rupp, L. J. (1996) 'Challenging Imperialism in International Women's Organizations, 1888–1945.' *NWSA Journal*, 8(1): 8.

Sachße, C. (1986) *Mütterlichkeit als Beruf: Sozialarbeit, Sozialreform und Frauenbewegung ; 1871–1929*. Frankfurt a. M.: Suhrkamp.

Sahlin, K., and L. Wedlin (2008) 'Circulating Ideas: Imitation, Translation and Editing.' In *The SAGE Handbook of Organizational Institutionalism*, edited by R. Greenwood, 218–42. Los Angeles: Sage Publications.

Said, E. W. (1983) 'Traveling Theory.' In *The World, the Text, and the Critic*, edited by E. W. Said, 226–47. Cambridge, MA: Harvard University Press.

Sassen, S. (2008) *Territory, authority, rights: from medieval to global assemblages*. Princeton, N.J.: Princeton Univ. Press.

Scherer, H. (2004) 'Die Auswirkungen von Besuchen deutscher sozialer Aktivisten im Londoner Settlement „Toynbee Hall" auf Entstehung und Konzeption der deutschen Nachbarschaftsheimbewegung.' *Rundbrief—Verband für Sozial-Kulturelle Arbeit e.V.* (2), http://jugendserver.spinnenwerk.de/~archiv/hits/2004_2_25.pdf. (accessed: Oct. 27, 2011).

Schreiber, A. (1904) 'Settlements. Ein Weg zum sozialen Verständnis.' *Sozialer Fortschritt—Hefte und Flugschriften für Volkswirtschaft und Sozialpolitik*, 23: 1–16.

Schüler, A. (2004) *Frauenbewegung und soziale Reform: Jane Addams und Alice Salomon im transatlantischen Dialog 1889–1933*. Stuttgart: Steiner.

Siegmund-Schultze, F. (1990) *Friedenskirche, Kaffeeklappe und die ökumenische Vision: Orig.-Ausg. ed. München 1910–1969*. Kaiser: Texte.

Star, S. L., and J. Griesemer (1989) 'Institutional Ecology, 'Translations,' and Boundary Objects: Amateurs and Professionals in Berkeley's Museum of Vertebrate Zoology, 1907–1939.' *Social Studies of Science*, 19: 387–420.

Strauss, A. L. (1993) *Continual Permutations of Action*. New York: Walter de Gruyter.

Treptow, R. (2004) 'Grenzüberschreitung und Globalisierung von Hilfe. Eine Skizze zur Internationalität Sozialer Arbeit.' In *International vergleichende soziale Arbeit: Sozialpolitik—Kooperation—Forschung*, edited by H. G. Homfeldt and K. Brandhorst, 10–24. Baltmannsweiler: Schneider-Verl. Hohengehren.

Treptow, R., and A. Walther. 2010. Internationalität und Vergleich in der Sozialen Arbeit. *Enzyklopädie Erziehungswissenschaft Online—Fachgebiet: Soziale Arbeit*, http://www.erzwissonline.de/fachgebiete/soziale_arbeit/beitraege/14100066.htm (accessed: Oct. 27, 2011).

Wendt, W. R. (2008) *Geschichte der sozialen Arbeit 1. Die Gesellschaft vor der sozialen Frage*. Stuttgart: Lucius & Lucius.

Westerkamp, A. (1917-1919) Aus amerikanischen Settlements: Briefe und Tagebuchbläter. Series of articles, published in: *Akademisch-Soziale Monatsschrift* 1–3.

Wietschorke, J. (2006) 'Soziales Settlement und ethnografisches Wissen. Zu einem Berliner Reformprojekt 1911–1933.' In *Grenzen & Differenzen: zur Macht sozialer und kultureller Grenzziehungen*, edited by T. Hengartner and J. Moser, 309–16. Leipzig: Leipziger Univ.-Verl.

Williams, R. (1973) 'Base and Superstructure in Marxist Cultural Theory.' *New Left Review*, I/82: 3–16.

Wimmer, A., and N. Glick Schiller (2002) 'Methodological Nationalism and Beyond: Nation-State Building, Migration and the Social Sciences.' *Global Networks*, 2(4): 301–34.

Zürn, M. (2003) 'Globalization and Global Governance: From Societal to Political Denationalization.' *European Review*, 11(3): 341–64.

# Contributors

**Désirée Bender**, Dipl. Päd., is a research associate at the Institute of Education, University of Mainz, Germany. Fields of interest: qualitative research, sociology of knowledge, transnationalism, discourse analysis, biography research, social support.

**Lothar Böhnisch** is a professor at the University of Dresden, Germany/Free University of Bolzano, Italy. Fields of interest: social work, gender (masculinity), social policy.

**Adrienne Chambon** is a professor at the Factor-Inwentash Faculty of Social Work, University of Toronto, Canada. Fields of interest: critical theory, arts and social work, history of social work, transnationalism.

**Arielle Dylan** is an assistant professor at the School of Social Work, St. Thomas University, Canada. Fields of interest: environmental social work and eco-justice, contemplative wellness practices, critical theory, relations between Aboriginal nations and the Crown in the Canadian context, international Roma experiences and community organising, transnationalism.

**Kay E. Ehlers** is a planner and social scientist in the City Administration of Hamburg, Germany. Fields of interest: concepts, management, and evaluation of (development) projects.

**Luann Good Gingrich** is an associate professor at the School of Social Work, Faculty of Liberal Arts & Professional Studies, York University Canada. Fields of interest: social exclusion and inclusion, transnational livelihoods, social policy and social welfare, intercultural/religious relations.

**Tina Hollstein**, Dipl. Päd., is a research associate at the Institute of Education, University of Mainz, Germany. Fields of interest: (illegal) migration, coping, transnationalism, social support, qualitative research.

**Lena Huber** is a PhD student and DFG scholarship holder at the Research Training Group "Transnational Social Support" at the Institute of Education, University of Mainz, Germany. Fields of interest: migration, poverty, coping, transnational social support, qualitative research (grounded theory and narrative analysis).

Stefan Köngeter, PhD, is a research fellow at the Faculty of Social Work, University of Toronto, Canada. Fields of interest: transnationalism, professionalisation of social work, child and youth care.

Ernie Lightman is a professor at the Faculty of Social Work, University of Toronto, Canada. Fields of interest: social policy.

Chin-ju Lin is an associate professor at the Graduate Institute of Gender Studies, Kaohsiung Medical University, Taiwan. Fields of interests: gender and ethnicity, family studies, intersectionality.

Wolfgang Schröer is a professor at the Institute of Social Pedagogy and Organisation Studies, University of Hildesheim, Germany. Fields of interest: transnational social work and social policy, child and youth care, history of social work and social policy.

Cornelia Schweppe is a professor at the Institute of Education, University of Mainz, Germany. Fields of interest: transnational and international social work, professionalisation of social work, poverty and social work, qualitative research methods, biography research, old age, social work in Latin America.

Wendy Smith is a senior lecturer at the Department of Management, Monash University, Australia. Fields of interest: discipline and area studies—social anthropology, management, Malaysian studies, Japanese studies, globalised new religious movements, management of religious diversity, social protection among Turkish migrants in Germany and Australia.

Elisabeth Tuider is a professor at the Faculty of Social Sciences, University of Kassel, Germany. Fields of interest: sociology of diversity, gender studies and feminist theory, qualitative research methods, migration research, Latin American studies, cultural and postcolonial studies.

Frank T. Y. Wang is an associate professor at the Graduate Institute of Social Work, National Chengchi University, Taipei, Taiwan. Fields of interest: aging, indigenous social work, long-term care.

Stephan Wolff is a professor at the Institute of Social Pedagogy and Organisation Studies, University of Hildesheim, Germany. Fields of interest: organisation studies, research methods, ethnomethodology, and conversation analysis.

# Index

T - #0173 - 071024 - C0 - 229/152/12 - PB - 9780415719728 - Gloss Lamination